D0912517

Multiple Choice Questions in Medicine

Multiple Choice Questions in Medicine

for the MRCP Examination (Part 1)

Patrick M. Bell MD, FRCP
Consultant Physician
Royal Victoria Hospital, Belfast

Brendan J. Collins BSc, MD, MRCP, FRACP
Consultant Gastroenterologist, Royal Perth Hospital
Clinical Associate Professor, University of Western Australia
(formerly Senior Lecturer, Queen's University of Belfast;
Consultant Physician, Royal Victoria Hospital, Belfast)

David R. McCluskey MD, FRCP
Senior Lecturer in Medicine, Queen's University of Belfast
Consultant Physician, Royal Victoria Hospital, Belfast

with a foreword by
A. H. G. Love

Third edition

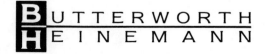

Butterworth-Heinemann Ltd
Linacre House, Jordan Hill, Oxford OX2 8DP

PART OF REED INTERNATIONAL BOOKS

OXFORD   LONDON   BOSTON
MUNICH   NEW DELHI   SINGAPORE   SYDNEY
TOKYO   TORONTO   WELLINGTON

First published by John Wright & Sons Ltd 1981
Second edition 1986
Third edition published by Butterworth-Heinemann 1992

British Library Cataloguing in Publication Data
Multiple Choice Questions in Medicine for
the MRCP Examination (Part 1). – 3rd ed.
  I. Bell, P. II. Collins, B. J.
  III. McCluskey, David R.
  610.76

ISBN 0 7506 0676 2

Typeset in 10 on 11pt Times by TecSet Ltd,
Wallington, Surrey

Printed and bound in Great Britain by
Biddles Ltd, Guildford and King's Lynn

Acknowledgements

In preparing this new edition many friends and colleagues, both knowingly and unknowingly, provided ideas for questions, and we thank them. We are particularly grateful to Dr P. McGarry (psychiatry) and Dr P. T. Jackson (paediatrics) for specialist help. Professor A. H. G. Love has been a source of encouragement and has kindly written the foreword. Widening the authorship from one to three for this edition has inflicted loss of recreational time—and occasionally temper—upon two more circles of family and friends. We thank them, and Mrs Frances Gallagher who typed it all, for being so understanding and patient with us.

Contents

Contents

Foreword

by A. H. G. LOVE
Professor and Chair, Department of Medicine,
the Queen's University of Belfast, and Director of Medicine,
Royal Victoria Hospital, Belfast

The demand for a third edition confirms the important place that this book occupies in the support material used by those preparing for the Membership. Its established position outlives the tenure of senior academic appointments. I am very pleased to endorse all the statements of my predecessor in forewords to previous editions.

The continuing strengths of the production lie in not only addressing model questions and answers which are educational in themselves, but also in refining teaching which is so important as an examination tool. The new edition maintains its excellent balance and is suitably updated to incorporate important areas of advances in medicine. I have no doubt that this new edition will enhance the likelihood of success of the diligent reader. Despite protestation in some circles, there is no evidence that a broadly based, refined and objective multiple choice question test will disappear in the foreseeable future. This book will remain excellent preparation for such tests.

Introduction

This book is designed for those taking the first part of the examination for membership of the Royal College of Physicians. It may also be of use to Final MB and other postgraduate students.

MRCP Part 1 is a 2½-hour examination consisting of 60 multiple choice questions each with five parts. It covers in detail a wide range of topics in internal medicine and basic science. To pass you must not only acquire sufficient knowledge, but also master the technique of doing multiple choice questions.

Acquiring the Knowledge

1. Plan your reading

Extensive reading is required, but remember that your time is limited. Your reading must be organised with some sort of time-table. Some candidates choose one of the large comprehensive textbooks of medicine and read it from cover to cover. Certainly most of the information is there, but it can be tedious. Others choose smaller monographs on the various topics. This is more interesting, but can mean using many different and expensive books.

Both these, as well as other, methods have been successfully used. Whatever method you decide upon, a little time spent planning your approach will be repaid.

2. Read widely

An examination consisting of 60 multiple choice questions can cover a wide range of subjects. Therefore you must read widely. Big subjects such as neurology and cardiology should be covered in depth. However, other subjects like tropical medicine and statistics also need some time spent on them. When all the questions from these other subjects are added together they form a significant percentage of the total paper. Also remember to read around the clinical cases that you encounter. Information gained in this way seems to be retained.

3. Know the basics

There is a widespread belief that MRCP Part 1 concentrates on the small print. While multiple choice questions lend themselves to testing fine detail, the extent of this is overestimated in the case of MRCP. The rare disorders do come up, but most questions are about common conditions. If one has time to read the small print it is better to know the rare manifestations of common conditions rather than the common manifestations of rare disorders.

While it is important to use modern textbooks, the examination does not test up-to-the-minute research developments. Stick to established and currently held dogma. Do not get so lost in learning facts that you forget underlying principles. A little time on applied physiology will be well spent.

Mastering the Technique

1. The scoring system

Each question contains a single statement followed by five possible completions. Any, none or all of the completed statements may be true. You can respond 'true', 'false' or 'don't know'. Each correct response receives one mark, and each incorrect response loses one mark. You receive a zero mark for each 'don't know'.

2. The marking system

You should study the instructions on marking the answer sheet issued by the colleges in their examination regulations.

The questions most people ask are 'What mark is needed to pass?', and 'On how many questions should I commit myself to a definite "true" or "false" when there is a risk of losing marks for wrong answers?'

No definite answer can be given to either question, but in general it is felt that a mark of above 60 per cent (or 180 out of 300) is needed to pass, remembering that the exact pass mark varies on each occasion that the examination takes place. There are two broad approaches used to achieve success.

The first approach is the cautious one and suggests that you mark 'true' or 'false' only those questions about which you are sure or nearly sure, and leave the rest as 'don't know'. Allowing for a few mistakes, if you commit yourself on about 210 parts, you would feel hopeful of passing, but remember you have virtually no chance if you answer fewer than 180 parts.

The more aggressive approach is based on the fact that guessing 'true' or 'false' gives a 50 per cent chance of being correct: an informed guess should have a better chance. Therefore it is claimed that by answering nearly all the questions, including those you are unsure about, you should do better than by being cautious. It is odd, though, how often informed guesses are incorrect!

Candidates have passed using either approach, and many probably fall between the two extremes. Much depends on your temperament. Try to work out which way is best for you while doing practice questions.

3. Practice
You must get practice with multiple choice questions. One selection is that released in book form by the colleges. All these questions have come up in previous papers and could come up again. Other questions available through correspondence courses vary in quality.

In doing practice questions you will see that certain subjects lend themselves to the multiple choice format. Try in your reading to focus on those pieces of information that could be easily included.

4. Ambiguous questions
Candidates constantly complain that certain questions are ambiguous, and of course in badly set papers this can be true. There is nothing more annoying than knowing the details of a particular question, but being unable to answer because of confused wording. In general things are improving and the MRCP Part 1 questions are of a high standard. Genuine ambiguity is rare. Remember that a fairly obvious answer is usually required. You can get into trouble by thinking too deeply.

Using this Book
The questions in this book are designed to be like those that you will see in the examination. We hope they will be helpful in revising the basic knowledge required, and in practising and developing the answering technique.

You are best to do them under examination conditions. Set yourself a given number of questions in the appropriate space of time. Do not look at the answers until you have finished.

The question format in this book is identical to that in the membership examination. The distribution of questions amongst the various subjects is roughly comparable, though up-to-date information on this is not available.

We hope the comments in the answer section will cope with some of the points that may arise. There is not enough space to deal with everything fully, but we believe that certain points are highlighted which, though important, are not given much space in the textbooks.

It is important that you realise why you have gone wrong in a particular question. Was it carelessness, a definite lack of factual knowledge or ignorance of basic principles? If you can answer these questions and go on to correct the deficiency, then this book may be of some help.

Finally, if there are answers with which after consideration you still disagree, we would like to hear from you. Then we may learn something as well!

Basic Sciences

1. **With regard to gene structure and function—**
   a. Non-coding DNA constitutes approximately 10 per cent of the human genome
   b. Reverse transcriptase facilitates synthesis of messenger RNA
   c. The DNA codon (coding unit) consists of four nucleotide bases
   d. Most amino acids are coded by more than one codon
   e. Translation is the process by which DNA chains serve as templates for complementary RNA molecules

2. **The median nerve supplies—**
   a. Brachioradialis
   b. Adductor pollicis
   c. Flexor carpi ulnaris
   d. Flexor pollicis brevis
   e. Palmar interossei

3. **Polymorphonuclear leucocytes—**
   a. Proliferate at inflammatory sites
   b. Are actively motile
   c. Produce immunoglobulin D
   d. Contain lysosomal granules
   e. Are involved in antigen presentation

4. **Galactose—**
   a. Has the same molecular weight as glucose
   b. Is directly converted to glucose by the enzyme galactose oxidase
   c. Is liberated when lactose is hydrolysed
   d. From the diet is stored in the liver as galactose-1-phosphate
   e. In the urine gives a positive test with Clinitest tablets

Answers overleaf

1. a. False Over 90 per cent
    b. False Facilitates synthesis of DNA from messenger RNA
    c. False Three nucleotide bases form a codon
    d. True   There are 64 possible coding combinations of three base pairs, and only 20 amino acids
    e. False This is transcription. Translation is the formation of polypeptide chains from RNA templates

2. a. False It is supplied by the radial nerve
    b. False It is supplied by the ulnar nerve
    c. False This and part of flexor digitorum profundus are the only flexors of the forearm supplied by the ulnar nerve. The median supplies the others
    d. True
    e. False

3. a. False After production in bone marrow they cannot proliferate
    b. True
    c. False Immunoglobulins are synthesised by plasma cells. Neutrophils are phagocytic cells
    d. True
    e. False Antigen presentation is primarily the role of macrophages

4. a. True   The only difference is the configuration of the radicals about one of the carbon atoms, i.e. they are epimers
    b. False Galactose first is converted to galactose-1-phosphate by galactokinase and then to glucose-1-phosphate by another enzyme
    c. True   Glucose is the other product liberated
    d. False It is converted to glucose-6-phosphate and can then be stored as glycogen. Galactose-1-phosphate accumulates in galactosaemia and causes liver damage
    e. True   It is a reducing sugar

5. **Characteristic effects of excessive noradrenaline include—**

   a. Increased total peripheral resistance
   b. Fall in diastolic blood pressure
   c. Less effect than adrenaline on bronchial smooth muscle
   d. Relaxation of anal and bladder sphincters
   e. Inhibition of muscle contraction in the pregnant uterus

6. **Factors that increase the oxygen content of blood at Po_2 of 50 mmHg (6.6 kPa) include an increase in—**

   a. pH
   b. Temperature
   c. Partial pressure of carbon dioxide
   d. 2,3-diphosphoglycerate
   e. Haemoglobin

7. **With regard to the blood supply of the heart—**

   a. The left coronary artery usually arises from the anterior aortic sinus
   b. The sinoatrial node is usually supplied by a branch of the left anterior descending artery
   c. The left coronary artery supplies the atrioventricular node
   d. The right coronary artery passes forward between the pulmonary trunk and the right atrium
   e. The marginal branch of the right coronary artery arises distal to the posterior interventricular branch

8. **In a normally distributed population—**

   a. The probability that an observation falls outside 1.96 standard deviations on either side of the mean is 0.01
   b. The mean, mode and median have the same value
   c. Calculation of the variance gives a measure of dispersion
   d. The standard deviation is calculated from the formula

$$\sqrt{\frac{\Sigma(x - \bar{x})}{n - 1}}$$

   e. The area under the curve within 2 standard deviations from the mean is constant, irrespective of the range of the observations

Answers overleaf

5. a. True   Due to its alpha effects
   b. False   This is the case with beta stimulation where the overall peripheral resistance is reduced
   c. True   Bronchodilation is a beta effect
   d. False   Both are constricted
   e. False   This is a beta effect and provides the rationale for the use of beta stimulators in preventing premature labour

6. a. True   This shifts the oxygen dissociation curve to the left
   b. False   This shifts the oxygen dissociation curve to the right
   c. False   This also shifts the curve to the right
   d. False   Again the curve is to the right. Hypoxia and acidosis tend to increase the levels of 2,3-diphosphoglycerate
   e. True

7. a. False   The left posterior aortic sinus
   b. False   55 per cent by the right coronary artery, 45 per cent by the left circumflex
   c. False   Usually the right coronary artery
   d. True
   e. False   It arises proximally

8. a. False   The probability of this is 5 per cent or 0.05
   b. True
   c. True   Standard deviation is the square root of the variance
   d. False   If this formula was used, negative and positive difference from the mean would cancel out. The correct formula is

$$\sqrt{\frac{\Sigma(x - \bar{x})^2}{n - 1}}$$

   e. True   It is this fact that enables generalisations about probability to be made

9. **The standard error of the mean—**

   a. Is calculated from the formula

   $$\frac{\text{standard deviation}}{n^2}$$

   b. Is an estimate of the standard deviation that would be obtained from the means of all possible samples of the given population
   c. Is independent of the variation in the population
   d. Is useful in studying the significance of the difference between the means of two samples
   e. Of a sample, drawn from a population which is not normally distributed, is of no value

10. **The tricarboxylic acid cycle (Krebs cycle)—**

   a. Is regulated by the concentration of oxaloacetate
   b. Takes place within the mitochondria
   c. Produces relatively more energy than does glycolysis for the equivalent amount of substrate
   d. Produces lactic acid as an important byproduct
   e. Provides substrates for amino acid synthesis

11. **Correlation—**

   a. Can be illustrated on a scatter diagram
   b. Represented by $r = 1$ implies a perfect positive linear correlation
   c. Represented by $r = 0.5$ implies that 50 per cent of the change in one variable can be accounted for by a change in the other variable
   d. Coefficients can have levels of significance attached which are independent of sample size
   e. Of high degree enables statements about causation to be made

Answers overleaf

9. a. False The formula is

$$\frac{\text{standard deviation}}{\sqrt{n}}$$

b. True
c. False The variation of the means of population samples will depend on the variability within the population
d. True
e. False The means of samples drawn from the population may form a normal distribution even where the population does not

10. a. True
b. True Whereas glycolysis takes place outside the mitochondria
c. True Breakdown to very simple molecules (carbon dioxide and water) causes a great release of energy
d. False This is a by-product of glycolysis
e. True For example alpha-ketoglutarate and succinate

11. a. True
b. True
c. False r^2 gives an estimate of this, i.e. $(0.5)^2 = 0.25$ or 25 per cent
d. False The significance can be estimated by using a t-test, and to attach a value of probability the degrees of freedom must be known
e. False Correlation is not causation

12. **In the proximal convoluted tubule—**

    a. About half the filtered uric acid is reabsorbed
    b. About 80 per cent of filtered water is reabsorbed under the influence of aldosterone
    c. Renin is produced
    d. Para-aminohippuric acid is actively reabsorbed
    e. Potassium is reabsorbed

13. **With regard to pathways in the spinal cord—**

    a. The sensations of pain and temperature appreciation are carried in the anterior spinothalamic tracts
    b. Fibres in the posterior (dorsal) columns terminate in the gracile and cuneate nuclei
    c. The posterior (dorsal) columns carry proprioceptive impulses from the contralateral side
    d. Most pyramidal tract fibres run in the lateral white columns of the cord
    e. The fasciculus gracilis is lateral to the fasciculus cuneatus

14. **Statistical tests that are non-parametric include—**

    a. Regression
    b. Correlation
    c. The Student's *t*-test
    d. Rank correlation
    e. Wilcoxon rank sum test

15. **Gastric acid production is increased by—**

    a. Hypoglycaemia
    b. Presence of food in the mouth
    c. Vasoactive intestinal polypeptide
    d. Acid in the duodenum
    e. Cholecystokinin-pancreozymin

Answers overleaf

12. a. False It is nearly all reabsorbed. Some is secreted in the distal convoluted tubule
    b. False This water is absorbed irrespective of the action of the aldosterone
    c. False It is produced in the juxtaglomerular apparatus
    d. False None is reabsorbed. Active secretion occurs in the distal tubule and its clearance gives an estimate of renal blood flow
    e. True

13. a. False Lateral spinothalamic tracts carry pain and temperature fibres
    b. True
    c. False Cross-over occurs in the medulla
    d. True
    e. False

14. a. False
    b. True Non-parametric tests are ones which can analyse data that are not normally distributed
    c. False Non-normally distributed data may be altered (e.g. by logarithms) so as to conform to a normal distribution and enable tests such as the *t*-test to be used
    d. True
    e. True

15. a. True Via a vagal reflex
    b. True Again via the vagus
    c. False The reverse is true
    d. False
    e. False

16. Cortisol—

    a. Increases margination of white blood cells
    b. Is required for excretion of a water load
    c. Release is mainly controlled by volume receptors in the great veins
    d. In excess gives pigmentation of the skin
    e. Has a plasma half-life of about 12 hours

17. In the *t*-test—

    a. An estimate of the probability that two samples come from the same population may be obtained
    b. In estimating the significance of the result the degrees of freedom must be known
    c. More than 30 observations are required before it can be used
    d. For a difference to be significant at a given probability, a higher value of *t* is required as the sample size increases
    e. The distribution of a variable in a sample can be compared with the distribution of that variable in another sample

18. The superior mesenteric artery—

    a. Arises at the level of the fourth lumbar vertebra
    b. Lies behind the pancreas at its origin
    c. Passes above the third part of the duodenum
    d. Supplies large intestine as far as the sigmoid colon
    e. Supplies the liver

19. Structures situated in the pons include the—

    a. Fourth nerve nucleus
    b. Vestibular nuclei
    c. Nucleus ambiguus
    d. Reticular formation
    e. Motor nucleus of the facial nerve

Answers overleaf

16. a. False Decreases margination of white blood cells
  b. True The water load test was commonly and sometimes dangerously used to diagnose Addison's disease
  c. False Adrenocorticotrophic hormone (ACTH) release from the pituitary is the main factor, and volume receptors have only a minor role in stimulating ACTH release
  d. False This is an ACTH effect
  e. False It is less than 2 hours

17. a. True
  b. True
  c. False The *t*-test is adapted for use with small samples
  d. False
  e. False The chi-squared test is used for this

18. a. False It arises at the level of the first lumbar vertebra
  b. True
  c. False It passes below
  d. False It supplies as far as the splenic flexure
  e. False The liver is supplied by the right and left hepatic arteries, which are branches of the coeliac artery

19. a. False It is in the midbrain
  b. True
  c. False It is in the medulla
  d. True
  e. True

20. Insulin—

    a. Is a glycoprotein

    b. Has a half-life in the circulation of 4 hours after intravenous injection

    c. Increases protein synthesis from amino acids in muscle

    d. Increases glucose uptake by the brain

    e. Increases the activity of glycogen phosphorylase

21. Tetraiodothyronine (T_4)—

    a. Synthesis is significantly reduced by standard doses of propranolol

    b. Concentrations in plasma are about twice those of tri-iodothyronine

    c. Is metabolised mainly by deiodination to form either tri-iodothyronine or reverse tri-iodothyronine

    d. In the protein bound form in plasma, is mostly attached to albumin

    e. Present in plasma as the free (non-protein bound) form represents about 10 per cent of total circulating tetraiodothyronine

22. Structures derived embryologically from the foregut include—

    a. Sigmoid colon

    b. First part of duodenum

    c. Lining of the bronchial tree

    d. Meckel's diverticulum

    e. Posterior pituitary

Answers overleaf

20. a. False It is a polypeptide with no carbohydrate component
    b. False The half-life is less than 20 minutes
    c. True
    d. False Insulin causes glucose uptake in muscle and adipose tissue but not in brain
    e. False Insulin increases the activity of the enzymes of glycogen synthesis

21. a. False
    b. False Concentrations of tri-iodothyronine are about 50 times less than those of tetraiodothyronine
    c. True
    d. False Most is bound to a specific thyroid binding globulin
    e. False About 0.05 per cent of total tetraiodothyronine is present in the free form

22. a. False The primitive endodermal foregut extends as far as the site of entry of the bile duct into the duodenum
    b. True
    c. True
    d. False Meckel's diverticulum is the vestige of the vitellointestinal duct
    e. False The anterior pituitary is derived from the primitive oral cavity (Rathke's pouch)

23. **Antibiotics that act predominantly by interference with the bacterial cell wall include—**

    a. Benzylpenicillin
    b. Trimethoprim
    c. Tetracycline
    d. Vancomycin
    e. Cephaloridine

24. **Viruses of which the nucleic acid core consists of DNA include—**

    a. Varicella-zoster virus
    b. Human immunodeficiency virus
    c. Adenovirus
    d. Poliovirus
    e. Influenza virus

25. **The glomerular filtration rate—**

    a. Is increased in patients with hypoproteinaemia
    b. Is equal to the rate of plasma flow to the glomerulus
    c. Is reduced in patients with chronic urinary retention
    d. Corresponds to the renal clearance of inulin
    e. Is directly proportional to systolic blood pressure

Answers overleaf

23. a. True Synthesis of cell wall mucopeptide is inhibited
   b. False Effect is by interference with folic acid metabolism
   c. False This also interferes with protein synthesis and prevents binding of transfer RNA to ribosomes
   d. True
   e. True The cephalosporins have a similar mode of action to the penicillins

24. a. True As are other members of the herpesvirus group, e.g. cytomegalovirus, Epstein–Barr virus and herpes simplex virus
   b. False
   c. True
   d. False The enteroviruses, of which poliovirus is one, are RNA viruses
   e. False The myxoviruses, of which influenza is one, are RNA viruses

25. a. True Decreased colloid osmotic pressure reduces glomerular filtration
   b. False Only 20–25 per cent of plasma is filtered
   c. True Due to increased pressure in Bowman's capsule
   d. True
   e. False Autoregulation ensures constant glomerular blood flow and filtration over a wide range of blood pressure

Cardiology

1. Recognised features of atrial myxoma include—

    a. Haemolytic anaemia
    b. Weight loss
    c. Pyrexia
    d. Syncopal attacks
    e. Progression to malignancy

2. Central cyanosis—

    a. Is a complication of treatment with dapsone
    b. Is present if the hands are blue and warm
    c. In those with right-to-left shunts can be completely corrected by inhalation of 100 per cent oxygen
    d. Is seen in normal people at altitudes of 1500 metres
    e. Is a feature of hereditary haemorrhagic telangiectasia

3. In the jugular venous pulse—

    a. Cannon 'a' waves occur with ventricular extrasystoles
    b. The 'a' wave is due to atrial contraction
    c. The 'x' descent is due to blood entering the ventricles
    d. The 'v' wave is prominent in constrictive pericarditis
    e. The 'y' descent is reduced in tricuspid stenosis

4. A fourth heart sound—

    a. Is usually physiological, when heard in those under 30 years old
    b. Corresponds in timing to the 'a' wave of the jugular venous pulse
    c. Is generated by forceful opening of the mitral valve
    d. Is associated with a reduction in ventricular compliance
    e. Is a recognised feature of systemic hypertension

Answers overleaf

1. a. True   Mechanical damage to red blood cells
    b. True   Constitutional features are common
    c. True
    d. True   The mobile tumour may cause mechanical obstruction
    e. False   The tumour is not locally invasive

2. a. True   May cause methaemoglobinaemia
    b. True   Peripheral cyanosis without central cyanosis implies cold, blue peripheries due to a poor circulation. If the circulation is good (i.e. the peripheries warm) and the hands are blue, central cyanosis must also be present
    c. False   Remember that in right-to-left shunts blood is bypassing the lungs and no amount of inspired oxygen can compensate
    d. False   Higher altitudes of around 4500 metres are required
    e. True   Pulmonary ateriovenous fistulas are found and these cause right-to-left shunting

3. a. True   If ventricular and atrial systole coincide
    b. True
    c. False   It is due to atrial relaxation and/or the downward movement of the tricuspid valve ring with the onset of ventricular systole
    d. False   While jugular venous pressure is increased the amplitude of the wave form is decreased
    e. True   The 'y' descent is due to blood filling the right ventricle from the right atrium. This filling is reduced in tricuspid stenosis

4. a. False   An audible fourth heart sound is generally pathological
    b. True   Both coincide with atrial contraction
    c. False   A fourth heart sound occurs late in diastole and is associated with rapid movement of blood into the ventricles
    d. True   Since the atrium must contract against greater ventricular resistance
    e. True   Since ventricular compliance is reduced

5. **The intensity of a murmur—**

   a. From the right side of the heart is increased by expiration
   b. Of aortic stenosis is increased by amyl nitrate
   c. Of hypertrophic obstructive cardiomyopathy is increased by Valsalva manoeuvre
   d. Of mitral stenosis is proportional to severity
   e. Of aortic incompetence is increased by hand-grip exercise

6. **Prominence of the main pulmonary arteries on chest X-ray may be seen in—**

   a. Ventricular septal defect
   b. Valvular pulmonary stenosis
   c. Fallot's tetralogy
   d. Severe mitral stenosis
   e. Multiple pulmonary emboli

7. **Constrictive pericarditis—**

   a. Characteristically produces acute pulmonary oedema
   b. Follows rheumatic fever
   c. Characteristically causes gross cardiomegaly on chest X-ray
   d. May be caused by rheumatoid arthritis
   e. Causes increased cardiac pulsation on fluoroscopy

8. **The electrocardiogram (ECG) in acute pulmonary embolism characteristically shows—**

   a. Sinus bradycardia
   b. ST and T wave changes in V_5 and V_6
   c. Left axis shift
   d. Changes which may disappear in a few days
   e. Right bundle branch block

9. **In pure mitral stenosis—**

   a. A third heart sound is heard
   b. The apex beat is displaced
   c. Infective endocarditis is a characteristic complication
   d. Women are affected more often than men
   e. Recurrent chest infections are an early feature

Answers overleaf

5. a. False Inspiration decreases intrathoracic pressure and causes blood to enter the right side of the heart

   b. True Amyl nitrate lowers peripheral resistance and increases the gradient between the left ventricle and aorta

   c. True The heart is made smaller and obstruction increased

   d. False The length of the murmur is proportional to severity

   e. True Hand-grip exercise increases peripheral resistance and therefore increases the gradient between the aorta and left ventricle in diastole

6. a. True Due to increased blood flow

   b. True Due to post-stenotic dilatation

   c. False The outflow obstruction is subvalvular and there is no post-stenotic dilatation. Blood flow through the pulmonary arteries is much reduced

   d. True Due to pulmonary hypertension

   e. True Again due to pulmonary hypertension

7. a. False

   b. False Virtually never happens

   c. False The constricted heart is often of normal size

   d. True With the decline of tuberculosis, this is now quite a common cause

   e. False The ventricular movement is reduced

8. a. False Sinus tachycardia is usual. Chest pain and sinus bradycardia suggest an inferior myocardial infarction

   b. False These changes are usually seen in the right ventricular leads

   c. False Right axis shift may occur

   d. True

   e. True

9. a. False A third heart sound is due to ventricular filling and this is impaired in mitral stenosis

   b. False Unless mitral incompetence is present

   c. False Incompetent valves are more often the seat of endocarditis

   d. True

   e. True

10. **Initial presentations of mitral valve prolapse (floppy mitral valve syndrome) include—**

    a. Mitral incompetence
    b. Chest pain
    c. Opening snap detected on routine auscultation
    d. Infective endocarditis
    e. Q waves and ST elevation on inferolateral chest leads on routine ECG

11. **The first heart sound is loud in—**

    a. First degree heart block
    b. Lown-Ganong-Levine syndrome
    c. Mitral stenosis with a heavily calcified valve
    d. Sinus bradycardia
    e. Hypertrophic obstructive cardiomyopathy

12. **Characteristic features of severe aortic stenosis are—**

    a. Exertional syncope
    b. Loud aortic second sound
    c. Blood pressure of 105/50 mmHg
    d. Early closure of the aortic valve
    e. Catheter gradient of 60 mmHg across the valve

13. **In hypertrophic obstructive cardiomyopathy—**

    a. Mitral incompetence may develop
    b. The murmur increases in intensity when the patient squats
    c. A family history is nearly always obtained
    d. Pregnancy is well tolerated
    e. Syncope is a characteristic symptom

14. **Characteristic features of Eisenmenger's syndrome complicating atrial septal defect include—**

    a. Development before 20 years of age
    b. Giant 'a' waves
    c. Pulmonary incompetence
    d. Differential cyanosis
    e. Necessity of surgical correction

Answers overleaf

10.
a. True   Severe mitral incompetence can occur rarely
b. True
c. False   A midsystolic click is characteristic
d. True   Many cardiologists recommend antibiotic prophy-laxis for surgical procedures
e. False   These findings suggest myocardial infarction

11.
a. False   The PR interval is long and the first heart sound varies inversely in intensity with the length of the PR interval
b. True   The PR interval is short
c. False   The heavily calcified valve cannot close rapidly enough to produce the classic loud first heart sound
d. False
e. False

12.
a. True   The cardiac output cannot increase in response to the increased demand during exercise
b. False   The aortic second sound should be soft
c. False   A low pulse pressure would be expected
d. False   Aortic valve closure is delayed and may cause 'reversed splitting'
e. True

13.
a. True   This probably results from distortion of the mitral valve by the hypertrophic left ventricle
b. False   On squatting venous return to the heart increases, the heart dilates and outflow obstruc-tion is reduced
c. False   This occurs in about 30 per cent of cases
d. True   A little surprising
e. True

14.
a. False   It usually occurs in later life
b. True   Due to pulmonary hypertension
c. True   Again due to pulmonary hypertension
d. False   Differential cyanosis (i.e. cyanosis of the lower part of the body more than the upper part of the body) is seen in Eisenmenger's syndrome compli-cating patent ductus
e. False   If the septal defect is closed an intolerable bur-den is placed on the right side of the heart

15. **A prolonged QT interval on ECG may be seen with—**
    a. Hypercalcaemia
    b. Digitalis therapy
    c. Ischaemic heart disease
    d. Hypothermia
    e. Amiodarone

16. **In left ventricular failure the following parameters are characteristically increased—**
    a. Pulmonary venous pressure
    b. Left ventricular end-diastolic pressure
    c. Lung compliance
    d. P_{O_2}
    e. P_{CO_2}

17. **In atrial fibrillation—**
    a. Cardiac output is reduced by approximately 10 per cent
    b. Atria contract at a rate of 350–600 per minute
    c. The ventricular rate is regular if there is coexistent complete heart block
    d. The sick sinus syndrome is a precipitating cause
    e. The intensity of the first heart sound is variable

18. **In infective endocarditis—**
    a. Due to fungal infection, surgical removal of the infected valve is often required
    b. In a drug addict, valve replacement is contraindicated
    c. A history of recent dental treatment is obtained in over half of all cases
    d. Affecting the right side of the heart, positive blood cultures are less likely
    e. Due to *Streptococcus bovis* infection, underlying colonic neoplasm may be found

19. **'Cannon waves' in the neck are a feature of—**
    a. Tricuspid stenosis
    b. Ventricular tachycardia
    c. Atrioventricular junctional (nodal) rhythm
    d. Right bundle branch block
    e. Atrial fibrillation

Answers overleaf

15. a. False The QT interval is short
     b. False Again here the QT interval is reduced
     c. True
     d. True
     e. True

16. a. True
     b. True
     c. False The oedematous lungs are harder to move
     d. False The Po_2 is reduced
     e. False Hyperventilation allows carbon dioxide to be excreted since it diffuses more easily across the alveolar membrane

17. a. False Loss of atrial contraction reduces cardiac output by 20–30 per cent
     b. False Atria do not contract at all
     c. True
     d. True The association of sinus node dysfunction and atrial tachyarrhythmia is called the 'brady–tachy' syndrome
     e. True

18. a. True
     b. False Surgical risks are not significantly greater than in non-addicts
     c. False Studies have shown that less than 20 per cent had dental treatment in the previous 3 months
     d. True
     e. True

19. a. False Large 'a' waves are a feature
     b. True There is dissociation between atrial and ventricular contraction
     c. True Complete heart block is the other cause
     d. False
     e. False

20. **In a patient with tachycardia of 170 beats per minute likely results of carotid sinus massage are—**

    a. Return to sinus rhythm if the original rhythm was rapid atrial fibrillation
    b. Gradual slowing towards normal if the original rhythm was ventricular tachycardia
    c. Temporary slowing if the original rhythm was sinus tachycardia
    d. Return to sinus rhythm if the original rhythm was paroxysmal atrial tachycardia
    e. No effect if the original rhythm was atrial flutter

21. **Reversed splitting of the second heart sound is a recognised feature of—**

    a. Pulmonary hypertension
    b. Wolff–Parkinson–White syndrome
    c. Aortic stenosis
    d. Left bundle branch block
    e. First degree heart block

22. **Features more suggestive of ventricular rather than atrial tachycardia with aberrant conduction include—**

    a. Variable intensity of the first heart sound
    b. Sudden slowing of heart rate following carotid sinus massage
    c. Occurrence of fusion beats
    d. Left axis deviation
    e. QRS complex greater than 140 ms

23. **Causes of a dominant R wave in lead V_1 include—**

    a. Right atrial hypertrophy
    b. Right bundle branch block
    c. Wolff–Parkinson–White syndrome type B
    d. Right ventricular hypertrophy
    e. True posterior myocardial infarction

Answers overleaf

20. a. False   Temporary slowing may occur but the rhythm remains irregular
    b. False   Usually no effect
    c. True
    d. True
    e. False   Slowing associated with increased atrioventricular block is common

21. a. False
    b. False   The first heart sound is sometimes loud due to the short PR interval
    c. True   Aortic valve closure is delayed and may follow pulmonary valve closure in expiration. Then in inspiration pulmonary valve closure is delayed and the degree of splitting may narrow
    d. True   Again aortic valve closure is delayed
    e. False   The first heart sound is soft

22. a. True
    b. False
    c. True   Intermittent conduction of an atrial beat results in fusion of sinus and tachycardia QRS
    d. False
    e. True   Bundle branch block accompanying supraventricular tachycardia does not usually widen the QRS complex to this degree

23. a. False   Tall, peaked P waves in V_1 are characteristic
    b. True   The characteristic RSR pattern helps distinguish this from other causes of tall R waves
    c. False   Dominant R waves in V_1 are a feature of the more usual type A
    d. True   May be associated right axis shift and sometimes right atrial hypertrophy
    e. True   The equivalent of the Q wave

24. Characteristic features of Wolff–Parkinson–White syndrome include—

a. Association with hypocalcaemia
b. Wide QRS complexes
c. 'Delta' waves on ECG during paroxysmal tachycardia
d. Ventricular fibrillation complicating atrial fibrillation
e. Reliable prevention of arrhythmia by digoxin

25. Oxygen therapy will significantly improve central cyanosis in—

a. Transposition of the great vessels
b. Mitral stenosis
c. Pulmonary fibrosis
d. Congestive cardiomyopathy
e. Methaemoglobinaemia

Answers overleaf

24. a. False
 b. True
 c. False Most often conduction during tachycardia is through the normal atrioventricular system producing normal QRS complexes
 d. True Atrial fibrillation requires prompt treatment
 e. False Digoxin is contraindicated

25. a. False Right-to-left shunting causes blood to bypass the lungs
 b. True
 c. True
 d. True
 e. False Cyanosis is not due to deoxygenated haemoglobin

Dermatology

1. Causes of scarring alopecia include—

a. Psoriasis
b. Discoid lupus
c. Severe iron deficiency anaemia
d. Lichen planus
e. Morphoea

2. Skin lesions associated with underlying malignant disease include—

a. Acquired ichthyosis
b. Acquired hypertrichosis lanuginosa
c. Lupus pernio
d. Erythema gyratum repens
e. Lichen planus

3. Characteristic features of pemphigus vulgaris include—

a. Highest incidence in old age
b. Subepidermal bullae
c. Mucosal involvement
d. Intense itch
e. Presence of autoantibody in skin

4. The Koebner phenomenon is a recognised feature of—

a. Dermatitis herpetiformis
b. Psoriasis
c. Acne vulgaris
d. Lichen planus
e. Molluscum contagiosum

5. Pitting of the fingernails is seen in—

a. Dermatitis herpetiformis
b. Psoriasis
c. Alopecia areata
d. Acne rosacea
e. Arsenic poisoning

Answers overleaf

1. a. False   Although the scalp is often involved, alopecia is rare and does not scar
   b. True   Scarring alopecia is typical
   c. False   Diffuse alopecia may be seen
   d. True
   e. True

2. a. True
   b. True
   c. False   A feature of sarcoidosis
   d. True
   e. False

3. a. False   It is a disease of middle age
   b. False   They are intraepidermal. In dermatitis herpetiformis and pemphigoid they are subepidermal
   c. True   Mucosal involvement is rare in dermatitis herpetiformis and pemphigoid
   d. False   Again unlike dermatitis herpetiformis
   e. True   This can be demonstrated by immunofluorescence. Serum antibodies are also present

4. a. False   The Koebner phenomenon is the induction at the site of trauma of skin changes present elsewhere
   b. True   It is particularly characteristic of psoriasis
   c. False
   d. True
   e. True

5. a. False
   b. True
   c. True
   d. False
   e. False   But horizontal white lines are found on the nails (Mees' lines)

6. Well-recognised side-effects of the retinoid etretinate include—

a. Hirsutism
b. Hyperostosis
c. Hypocalcaemia
d. Onycholysis
e. Hypertriglyceridaemia

Answers overleaf

6. a. False Diffuse hair loss may occur. Dryness of skin and
mucous membranes is common
b. True
c. False Hypercalcaemia is an occasional feature
d. True
e. True

Endocrinology and Metabolic Diseases

1. **Recognised findings in acromegaly include—**

   a. Hypertension
   b. Increased perspiration
   c. Hyperprolactinaemia
   d. Hypophosphataemia
   e. Cardiomyopathy

2. **In a 50-year-old woman suspected of having panhypopituitarism features that would be characteristic of this diagnosis include—**

   a. Pale skin and a haemoglobin level of 6.0 g/dl
   b. History of failure to lactate after last child
   c. Potassium concentration of 2.0 mmol/l
   d. Absent body hair
   e. Obesity

3. **Drugs that cause goitre include—**

   a. Carbimazole
   b. Digoxin
   c. Lithium
   d. Iodine
   e. Rifampicin

4. **Symptomatic hypoglycaemia is a recognised feature of—**

   a. von Gierke's disease
   b. Renal glycosuria
   c. Acute alcoholic intoxication
   d. Phenylketonuria
   e. Primary hepatoma

5. **Necrobiosis lipoidica diabeticorum—**

   a. Is more common in females than males
   b. Is usually painful
   c. Is characteristically yellow in the centre due to lipid deposition
   d. Typically affects one limb
   e. Often improves after a prolonged period of careful metabolic control of diabetes

Answers overleaf

1. a. True
    b. True
    c. True   May be seen in some patients
    d. False Hyperphosphataemia is seen occasionally
    e. True   Is an important cause of death

2. a. False Pallor without anaemia is characteristic of hypo-pituitarism. If anaemia occurs it is mild
    b. True   This would suggest postpartum haemorrhage leading to pituitary necrosis as the cause
    c. False
    d. True
    e. False Asthenia is common

3. a. True   Most goitrogens block thyroid hormone synthesis. The gland hypertrophies to maintain the euthyroid state. This is said to be mediated by thyroid stimulating hormone (TSH), but is in fact elevated only occasionally
    b. False
    c. True
    d. True
    e. False

4. a. True   Glucose-6-phosphatase is deficient
    b. False Renal losses are small
    c. True   Beware of correction of hypoglycaemia without giving vitamin supplements, as Wernicke's encephalopathy can be precipitated
    d. False
    e. True   A variety of fibromas and sarcomas also cause hypoglycaemia. Insulin-like growth factors may be responsible in some cases

5. a. True
    b. False
    c. True
    d. False Usually bilateral affecting both lower legs
    e. False A few cases improve spontaneously, but blood glucose control does not seem to be important

6. Recognised features of thyrotoxicosis include—

   a. Deafness
   b. Pretibial myxoedema
   c. Ataxic gait
   d. Glycosuria
   e. Unilateral exophthalmos

7. Features of hypothyroidism due to primary involvement of the thyroid gland include—

   a. No rise in TSH levels in response to intravenous thyrotrophin releasing hormone (TRH)
   b. Megaloblastic anaemia
   c. Reduced thyroid binding globulin concentration
   d. Increased creatine phosphokinase concentration (CPK)
   e. Delta waves on ECG

8. In Paget's disease—

   a. There is characteristically an increase in bone resorption and formation
   b. Bones are stronger than normal
   c. Dysarthria is a recognised complication
   d. High-output cardiac failure is a common cause of death
   e. Urinary hydroxyproline excretion is increased

9. Causes of hypercalcaemia include—

   a. Nifedipine
   b. Sarcoidosis
   c. Osteoporosis
   d. Thyrotoxicosis
   e. Frusemide

Answers overleaf

6. a. False A feature of hypothyroidism
    b. True And is especially associated with exophthalmos and a high level of thyroid stimulating immuno-globulin
    c. False
    d. True
    e. True Although retro-orbital tumours need to be considered

7. a. False The hypothalamopituitary axis is responsive to TRH and high TSH levels are produced, unlike hyperthyroidism and hypopituitarism
    b. False Peripheral blood macrocytosis occurs without megaloblastic change in the marrow
    c. False
    d. True A myopathy is seen occasionally, while a raised CPK level is quite common
    e. False These are seen in Wolff–Parkinson–White syndrome

8. a. True
    b. False Although bones may be thicker they are weaker than usual. Pathological fractures are a complication
    c. True Due to brain stem compression
    d. False It is quite rare
    e. True As in other disorders where bone breakdown allows hydroxproline release from collagen matrix

9. a. False
    b. True The mechanism is thought to be increased vitamin D sensitivity
    c. False Serum calcium, phosphate and alkaline phosphatase levels should all be normal
    d. True It is a rare complication
    e. False The thiazide diuretics may cause hypercalcaemia, but the loop diuretics cause increased calcium excretion

10. **Osteoporosis—**

    a. Causes Looser's zones
    b. May complicate thyrotoxicosis
    c. Is associated with a raised alkaline phosphatase concentration
    d. Results from long-term use of heparin
    e. Characteristically produces continuous bone pain

11. **Hypocalcaemia is found in association with—**

    a. Acute pancreatitis
    b. Hypomagnesaemia
    c. Hysterical overbreathing
    d. Cushing's syndrome
    e. Pseudohypoparathyroidism

12. **Hypercholesterolaemia—**

    a. Is usually caused by deficiency of the enzyme lipoprotein lipase
    b. May present with arthritis
    c. Of severe degree is inherited as a dominant trait
    d. Is reversed by administration of bile salts
    e. Is a characteristic feature of primary biliary cirrhosis

13. **Recognised features of hyperparathyroidism include—**

    a. Normal alkaline phosphatase levels
    b. Metabolic alkalosis
    c. Hyperphosphaturia
    d. Increased blood urea concentration
    e. Increased urinary hydroxyproline concentration

14. **Features of Cushing's syndrome due to ectopic ACTH production that help to differentiate from Cushing's syndrome due to a basophil adenoma include—**

    a. Hyperglycaemia
    b. Marked hypokalaemia
    c. Suppression of cortisol after dexamethasone 2 mg 6-hourly for 2 days
    d. Males most commonly affected
    e. Grossly elevated ACTH levels

    Answers overleaf

10. a. False   They are found in osteomalacia
    b. True
    c. False
    d. True   Though this is not a very common situation
    e. False   The pain is typically intermittent and associated with fractures. Osteomalacia produces continuous pain

11. a. True
    b. True   Another important cause is chronic renal failure
    c. False   This causes alkalosis and hence tetany by lowering the ionised calcium level, but the total calcium level (ionised and protein bound) is unaltered and this is what is usually measured
    d. False   Hypercalciuria is occasionally seen
    e. True   By end-organ insensitivity to parathormone

12. a. False   Lipoprotein lipase deficiency is responsible for hyperchylomicronaemia which is rare
    b. True
    c. True
    d. False   Cholestyramine which binds cholesterol-containing bile salts is used
    e. True

13. a. True   The raised alkaline phosphatase level reflects bone disease which is not always present
    b. False   There is a tendency towards hyperchloraemic acidosis
    c. True   Parathormone increases phosphate excretion
    d. True   Renal failure may occur due to nephrocalcinosis
    e. True

14. a. False   It occurs in both
    b. True   In most cases of Cushing's syndrome hypokalaemia is mild but it can be severe in ectopic ACTH production
    c. False   Ectopic ACTH production does not suppress in the high-dose dexamethasone suppression test, while cortisol production is suppressed in Cushing's due to a basophil adenoma
    d. True   Related to the higher incidence of oat cell carcinoma in males
    e. True   ACTH levels are much less markedly elevated in a basophil adenoma

15. Characteristic features of carcinoma of the thyroid include—

a. History of treatment of hyperthyroidism with radioactive iodine
b. Increased uptake of iodine in the cancerous area as shown by a thyroid scan
c. Hypocalcaemia in the medullary type
d. Normal serum thyroxine levels
e. Benefit from thyroxine in papillary type

16. In phaeochromocytoma—

a. Treatment of choice for an acute hypertensive episode is intravenous beta-blockade
b. Distant metastases are often present at the time of diagnosis
c. Paroxysmal hypotension is recognised
d. There is an excess of 5-hydroxyindoleacetic acid in the urine
e. A family history of the disease may be obtained

17. Pituitary diabetes insipidus is improved by—

a. Water restriction
b. Glucagon
c. Lithium
d. Chlorpropamide
e. Chlorothiazide

18. Recognised features of Conn's syndrome include—

a. Low urinary potassium levels
b. Tetany
c. High plasma renin levels
d. Reduced sweat levels of sodium
e. U waves on ECG

19. In excessive antidiuretic hormone secretion—

a. Tetracycline therapy may be the cause
b. A history of head injury may be obtained
c. Plasma osmolarity is increased
d. Urinary sodium excretion is low
e. Ankle oedema is characteristic

Answers overleaf

15. a. False   No such association is proved
      b. False   Hot nodules are nearly always benign
      c. False   Although calcitonin tends to lower calcium levels, hypocalcaemia is rarely seen
      d. True
      e. True   Thyroxine is of less benefit in the other types

16. a. False   A beta-blocker alone allows uncontrolled alpha effects
      b. False   Less than 10 per cent of tumours are malignant
      c. True   Probably in those cases where adrenaline, with its vasodilator effects, is in excess
      d. False   It is adrenaline, noradrenaline and their derivatives that are found
      e. True   As may a history in the patient or family of multiple endocrine neoplasia type II, neurofibromatosis or cerebellar haemangioblastoma

17. a. False   Water restriction and the failure of urine to concentrate is diagnostic but not therapeutic
      b. False
      c. False   Lithium causes diabetes insipidus
      d. True   Hypoglycaemia is a troublesome complication
      e. True   Is also useful in nephrogenic diabetes insipidus

18. a. False
      b. True   Due to alkalosis
      c. False   They are low
      d. True   As with urine
      e. True   Due to hypokalaemia

19. a. False   Demeclocycline may be used in treatment
      b. True   Various intracranial disorders, e.g. trauma, infection and neoplasm, are among the many causes of this syndrome
      c. False   Haemodilution occurs
      d. False   Sodium excretion is not fundamentally affected
      e. False   Despite the water overload, oedema is unusual

20. Glycosuria is a recognised finding in—

    a. Acute intermittent porphyria
    b. Wilson's disease
    c. Hypothyroidism
    d. Galactosaemia
    e. Subarachnoid haemorrhage

21. Hyperprolactinaemia is a recognised finding in—

    a. Chlorpromazine therapy
    b. Amphetamine therapy
    c. Hyperthyroidism
    d. Levodopa therapy
    e. Chromophobe adenoma

22. Causes of hirsutism include—

    a. Addison's disease
    b. Adrenal carcinoma
    c. Thyrotoxicosis
    d. Phenytoin
    e. Polycystic ovary syndrome

23. Causes of low urinary calcium include—

    a. Renal tubular acidosis
    b. Cushing's syndrome
    c. Chronic glomerulonephritis
    d. Osteomalacia
    e. Paget's disease

24. Increased radioactive iodine uptake by the thyroid is characteristic of—

    a. Factitious hyperthyroidism
    b. Subacute thyroiditis
    c. Iodine deficiency
    d. Graves' disease
    e. Patients taking carbimazole

Answers overleaf

20. a. False
b. True   Due to renal tubular defect
c. False
d. False   Reducing sugar as galactose is detected in the urine, but not glucose
e. True

21. a. True   Chlorpromazine is a dopamine antagonist
b. False   Prolactin secretion is suppressed
c. False   Hyperprolactinaemia is a feature of hypothyroidism
d. False
e. True   Prolactin-secreting tumours are often chromophobic on routine stains

22. a. False
b. True   And may also cause Cushing's syndrome
c. False   But it does occasionally cause gynaecomastia
d. True   A reason for avoiding its use in adolescent females
e. True

23. a. False   Hypercalciuria is usual. Calculi may occur
b. False   Hypercalciuria is occasionally seen
c. True
d. True
e. False   Hypercalciuria may be seen

24. a. False   Exogenous hormone suppresses iodine uptake
b. False   The hyperthyroidism sometimes seen is thought to represent release of hormone from damaged cells, rather than increased iodine uptake and hormone synthesis
c. True
d. True
e. False   Carbimazole suppresses iodine uptake

25. Characteristic features of Wilson's disease include—

    a. Raised serum copper levels
    b. Aminoaciduria
    c. Autosomal dominant inheritance
    d. Onset in the first year of life
    e. Haemolytic anaemia

Answers overleaf

25.
a. False It is low due to low levels of the binding protein caeruloplasmin
b. True Phosphate is also lost in the urine and may lead to bone disease
c. False It is recessive
d. False Between 6 and 20 years would be typical
e. True

Gastroenterology

1. **Causes of malabsorption include—**

   a. Levodopa therapy
   b. Immunoglobulin A deficiency
   c. Whipple's disease
   d. Methotrexate therapy
   e. High-density lipoprotein deficiency (Tangier disease)

2. **In achalasia of the oesophagus—**

   a. Presentation before the age of 20 years is usual
   b. Recurrent chest infections are characteristic
   c. Normal barium swallow excludes diagnosis
   d. Nifedipine worsens dysphagia
   e. Absence of oesophageal peristalsis is typical

3. **Reduced lower oesophageal sphincter tone is caused by—**

   a. Smoking
   b. Pregnancy
   c. Metoclopramide
   d. Systemic sclerosis
   e. Ingestion of a fatty meal

4. **An increased incidence of small bowel lymphoma is seen in patients with—**

   a. Congenital intestinal lymphangiectasia
   b. Coeliac disease
   c. Nodular lymphoid hyperplasia
   d. Eosinophilic gastroenteropathy
   e. Hepatic cirrhosis

5. **In the management of ulcerative colitis—**

   a. Sulphasalazine is reserved for the acute exacerbation
   b. Colectomy generally leaves systemic complications un-altered
   c. Steroids prevent relapse
   d. Pregnancy is best avoided while the disease is quiescent
   e. Regular B_{12} supplements are needed

Answers overleaf

1. a. False
  b. True   Through association with giardiasis, coeliac disease and food hypersensitivity
  c. True
  d. True
  e. False   Malabsorption does occur with abetalipoproteinaemia

2. a. False   Usually the third and fourth decade
  b. True   Due to aspiration
  c. False   May be normal in the early stages
  d. False   May help by relaxing the lower oesophageal sphincter
  e. True

3. a. True
  b. True   A factor in the heartburn of pregnancy
  c. False   May be beneficial in the treatment of reflux oesophagitis
  d. True
  e. True

4. a. False
  b. True
  c. True   An occasional complication of late onset hypogammaglobulinaemia
  d. False
  e. False

5. a. False   It is particularly useful in preventing relapse
  b. False   Joint and (particularly) skin and eye complications may all be helped. Note that sacroilitis generally is not helped
  c. False
  d. False   There is a slight risk of relapse, but usually pregnancy is well tolerated
  e. False B_{12} is absorbed normally, unlike Crohn's terminal ileitis

6. **Aetiological factors in acute pancreatitis include—**

   a. Addison's disease
   b. Hyperparathyroidism
   c. Hypothermia
   d. Pancreatic carcinoma
   e. Hyperlipidaemia

7. **In a patient with longstanding liver cirrhosis, factors that suggest the possibility of liver cell carcinoma include—**

   a. Splenomegaly
   b. Development of an arterial bruit over the liver
   c. High titre of antimitochondrial antibody
   d. A sudden increase in the alkaline phosphatase level
   e. Ascites with a protein content of 40 g/l

8. **Breath hydrogen tests—**

   a. Detect bacterial overgrowth in the colon
   b. Allow assessment of oral–caecal transit time
   c. Are characteristically abnormal in blind loop syndrome
   d. Are unhelpful in assessing lactose malabsorption
   e. Are contraindicated during pregnancy

9. **Malabsorption of pancreatic origin is characterised by—**

   a. Iron deficiency anaemia
   b. High faecal fat content
   c. High urinary indican
   d. Inability to absorb medium-chain triglyceride
   e. Low serum folate levels

10. **Characteristic features of ischaemic colitis at the onset of an attack include—**

    a. Inflamed rectal mucosa
    b. Normal barium enema
    c. Necessity of emergency surgery
    d. Signs of generalised peritonitis
    e. Bloody diarrhoea

Answers overleaf

6. a. False
    b. True
    c. True
    d. True   Acute pancreatitis in the elderly should raise this possibility
    e. True   Particularly hypertriglyceridaemia

7. a. False
    b. True   An arterial bruit usually indicates hepatoma or acute alcoholic hepatitis
    c. False   This is a feature of primary biliary cirrhosis
    d. True   Due to tumour obstructing the biliary tree
    e. True   Complicating peritonitis would also give an exudate

8. a. False   The normal colon has a heavy bacterial load
    b. True   Lactulose is used for this assessment
    c. True   An early rise in breath hydrogen reflects small bowel bacterial overgrowth
    d. False   The lactose breath hydrogen test is diagnostic
    e. False   No radioisotope is required

9. a. False   Iron is absorbed in the acid environment of the duodenum as usual
    b. True   The grossest degrees of steatorrhoea are seen in pancreatic malabsorption
    c. False
    d. False   A useful treatment option
    e. False B_{12} and folate are absorbed normally

10. a. False   The rectum is rarely involved
     b. False   The 'thumbprint' sign due to mucosal oedema is characteristic
     c. False   Conservative management is usually adequate
     d. False   This would be unusual
     e. True

11. **Recognised features of coeliac disease include—**

    a. Mouth ulcers
    b. Presentation some months after partial gastrectomy
    c. Hypersplenism
    d. IgA deposition in the dermis
    e. Family history of the disease

12. **Recognised complications of large intestinal diverticular disease include—**

    a. Blind loop syndrome
    b. Polyarthritis
    c. Massive bleeding
    d. Liver abscess
    e. Fistula formation

13. **In haemochromatosis—**

    a. Hepatoma complicates more often than in alcoholic cirrhosis
    b. Chondrocalcinosis is a recognised feature
    c. Total iron binding capacity is elevated
    d. Desferrioxamine is the treatment of choice
    e. Cardiac failure is the main cause of death in untreated cases

14. **There is a recognised association between duodenal ulceration and—**

    a. Intracranial injury
    b. Pernicious anaemia
    c. Renal failure
    d. Diabetes mellitus
    e. *Helicobacter* gastritis

15. **In severe pyloric stenosis findings include—**

    a. Hypokalaemia
    b. Raised urea level
    c. Low urinary pH
    d. Hypochloraemia
    e. Tetany

Answers overleaf

11.
a. True
b. True A subclinical defect may be exposed
c. False Splenic atrophy is characteristic
d. True A feature of both coeliac disease and dermatitis herpetiformis
e. True

12.
a. False
b. False Unlike ulcerative colitis, Crohn's disease and some infective diarrhoea
c. True
d. True Due to portal pyaemia
e. True

13.
a. True A significant cause of death in treated cases
b. True
c. False Iron binding is saturated
d. False Venesection is a quicker way of removing iron
e. True Liver complications such as encephalopathy and oesophageal varices are less common than in other types of cirrhosis

14.
a. True So-called 'Cushing's ulcer' may occur in the duodenum as well as in the stomach
b. False Hypochlorhydria prevails
c. True Gastrin excretion may be impaired
d. False
e. True

15.
a. True
b. True
c. True Despite systemic alkalosis, the sodium-retaining mechanisms at the distal tubule take precedence, and with potassium levels already low, hydrogen ions are excreted in exchange for sodium
d. True
e. True Due to alkalosis

16. **Characteristic features of Zollinger–Ellison syndrome include—**

    a. Diarrhoea
    b. Grossly exaggerated gastric acid response to intravenous pentagastrin
    c. Failure of cimetidine to ameliorate symptoms
    d. Benign behaviour of the pancreatic tumour
    e. Association with other endocrine tumours

17. **In a patient with liver cirrhosis, factors pointing towards an alcoholic aetiology include—**

    a. Peripheral neuropathy
    b. Raised serum IgM concentrations
    c. Parotid enlargement
    d. Macronodular cirrhosis
    e. Pancreatic calcification

18. **Characteristic features of the Budd–Chiari syndrome of hepatic vein obstruction include—**

    a. Association with polycythaemia vera
    b. Giant 'v' waves in the jugular venous pulse
    c. Generalised reduction of isotope uptake on technetium scanning
    d. Ascites
    e. Liver biopsy showing cirrhosis

19. **Recognised features of vitamin C deficiency include—**

    a. Macrocytosis
    b. Pigmented rash on the light-exposed areas
    c. Perifollicular haemorrhages
    d. Heart failure
    e. Osteoporosis

20. ***Helicobacter pylori—***

    a. Is a urease-producing organism
    b. Is more commonly present in the duodenum than in the stomach
    c. Stimulates a humoral antibody response
    d. Is a cause of hypochlorhydria
    e. Infection is found more commonly in children than in adults

    Answers overleaf

16. a. True   Acid in the duodenum inactivates lipase leading to fat malabsorption
     b. False   The acid output is already high due to high resting gastrin levels, and the exogenous pentagastrin makes little difference
     c. False   Adequate doses are often very effective
     d. False   Although slowly growing, they are most often malignant
     e. True   Especially parathyroid and pituitary

17. a. True   Thiamine deficiency in alcoholics commonly causes this
     b. False   Increased IgA is characteristic
     c. True   Probably reflects malnutrition
     d. False   Alcoholic cirrhosis is usually micronodular
     e. True   Alcohol-associated pancreatitis

18. a. True   And also with other thrombotic disorders
     b. False   The jugular venous pulse is dissociated from the liver by the obstruction. Hepatojugular reflux is negative. Giant 'v' waves are a feature of tricuspid incompetence
     c. False   Classically there is more prominent uptake centrally over the caudate lobe, because it drains separately into the inferior vena cava
     d. True
     e. False   Gross hepatic venous congestion dominates

19. a. True
     b. False   This is typical of pellagra
     c. True
     d. False   This is typical of beriberi
     e. True   Impaired formation of bone matrix

20. a. True   Detection of this urease forms the basis of a test for the organism
     b. False
     c. True   Serological tests have been developed that reliably confirm *Helicobacter pylori* infection
     d. True   May cause transient hypochlorhydria in the course of acute infection
     e. False

21. Major resection of the terminal ileum is associated with—

    a. Folic acid deficiency
    b. Sodium and water secretion by colonic mucosa
    c. Rapid fall in serum B_{12} levels
    d. Increased risk of biliary colic
    e. Uric acid renal stones

22. Colonic adenomatous polyps—

    a. Are present in approximately 5 per cent of the population over 65 years old
    b. Are the premalignant lesion in the majority of cases of colonic cancer
    c. Are usually asymptomatic
    d. Are a complication of longstanding ulcerative colitis
    e. Require laparotomy for removal

23. *Campylobacter jejuni* or *Campylobacter coli* infection in humans—

    a. Is caused by a gram-negative bacillus
    b. Spreads rapidly from person to person
    c. Produces clinical illness due to toxin formation
    d. Is usually responsive to erythromycin
    e. Produces sigmoidoscopic features indistinguishable from ulcerative colitis

24. Granuloma formation in the liver is a recognised feature of—

    a. Chronic active hepatitis
    b. Brucellosis
    c. Berylliosis
    d. Hodgkin's disease
    e. Leptospirosis

Answers overleaf

21.
  a. False Absorbed in the proximal small intestine
  b. True Bile salts enter the colon and stimulate sodium and water secretion
  c. False Stores of B_{12} in the liver prevent a fall in serum B_{12} levels for several years after resection
  d. True Due to cholesterol gallstones in bile salt deficient, lithogenic bile
  e. False But oxalate stones may occur

22.
  a. False They are much more common (around 30 per cent) in this age group
  b. True The adenoma–carcinoma sequence is well established
  c. True But occasionally bleed, or cause diarrhoea or intussusception
  d. False Pseudopolyps are not adenomatous. Cancer complicating ulcerative colitis arises from dysplastic mucosa
  e. False Most polyps can be safely removed at colonoscopy

23.
  a. True
  b. False Infection is usually acquired by eating contaminated food
  c. False Causes an invasive type of infection primarily of the small bowel but occasionally of the colon
  d. True Most cases resolve without antibiotic treatment
  e. True

24.
  a. False
  b. True Also true of other infections including tuberculosis, histoplasmosis and occasionally glandular fever
  c. True Due to industrial exposure. Sarcoidosis has several features in common including the presence of liver granulomas
  d. True Often subclinical
  e. False

25. Features more suggestive of Crohn's disease than ulcerative colitis include—

a. Granuloma formation
b. Pseudopolyp formation
c. Crypt abscesses
d. Sparing of the rectum
e. Attachment of affected bowel to adjacent viscera

Answers overleaf

25. a. True   But they may be absent
 b. False   Typical of ulcerative colitis. Pseudopolyps are islands of mucosa left by denudation of the surrounding mucosa
 c. False   Again typical of ulcerative colitis
 d. True   The rectum is always involved in ulcerative colitis
 e. True   This may lead to fistula formation

Haematology

1. **In a patient newly diagnosed as having chronic myeloid leukaemia, characteristic features would include—**

   a. Thrombocytopenia
   b. Basophilia
   c. Reduced leucocyte alkaline phosphatase
   d. Low B_{12} levels
   e. Elevated uric acid levels

2. **Disorders in which there is an abnormal amino acid substitution in the haemoglobin polypeptide chain include—**

   a. Paroxysmal nocturnal haemoglobinuria
   b. Methaemoglobinaemia
   c. Sickle cell trait
   d. Glucose-6-phosphate dehydrogenase deficiency
   e. Alpha-thalassaemia

3. **A myeloid type of leukaemoid reaction is recognised with—**

   a. Subphrenic abscess
   b. Carcinoma of the lung with bone metastases
   c. Infectious mononucleosis
   d. Acute haemolysis
   e. Whooping cough

4. **Indications for splenectomy include—**

   a. Polycythaemia vera
   b. Chronic idiopathic thrombocytopenic purpura
   c. Autoimmune haemolytic anaemia
   d. Sickle cell disease
   e. Pernicious anaemia

Answers overleaf

1. a. False Normal or increased platelet numbers are present in the early stages
   b. True
   c. True It may increase at the stage of blast cell transformation
   d. False Characteristically elevated
   e. True Due to increased cell turnover, although clinical gout is not a common presenting feature

2. a. False A red cell membrane defect is the problem
   b. False This is where haem is oxidised to the ferric state, and is usually induced by drugs or chemicals
   c. True Valine is substituted for glutamic acid at the sixth position of the beta chain
   d. False
   e. False Due to the failure of synthesis of alpha chains, gamma and beta chains are present in excess, but this is not the result of amino acid substitution

3. a. True As with other infections producing a profound neutrophil leucocytosis
   b. True
   c. False The blood picture is more likely to be confused with lymphatic leukaemia
   d. True
   e. False A marked lymphocytosis may be seen

4. a. False
   b. True Though splenomegaly is not prominent
   c. True The spleen is usually the main site of red blood cell destruction
   d. False The spleen is usually atrophic as a result of multiple infarcts
   e. False Splenomegaly, which is found in less than 10 per cent of cases, subsides with adequate replacement

5. **Haemolytic disorders in which haemolysis is characteristically intravascular include—**

   a. Beta-thalassaemia
   b. Hereditary spherocytosis
   c. Paroxysmal nocturnal haemoglobinuria
   d. Blackwater fever
   e. Pyruvate kinase deficiency

6. **Characteristic features of chronic idiopathic thrombocytopenic purpura include—**

   a. Females more often affected than males
   b. Bleeding into joints
   c. Splenomegaly
   d. Decreased number of megakaryocytes in the bone marrow
   e. Prolonged bleeding time

7. **Increased serum iron concentration is a feature of—**

   a. Anaemia due to chronic infection
   b. Thalassaemia
   c. Sideroblastic anaemia
   d. von Willebrand's disease
   e. Pernicious anaemia

8. **A dimorphic blood picture is a feature of—**

   a. Sideroblastic anaemia
   b. Malabsorption
   c. Thalassaemia
   d. Recent blood transfusion
   e. Aplastic anaemia

Answers overleaf

5. a. False
   b. False Extravascular haemolysis is usual with red cells being destroyed in the spleen
   c. True The classic case of intravascular haemolysis. It also occurs in heart valve haemolysis, mismatched transfusions, infections, burns and sometimes in autoimmune haemolytic anaemia and glucose-6-phosphate dehydrogenase deficiency
   d. True *Clostridium welchii* septicaemia is the other typical infective cause
   e. False

6. a. True In the acute type sex incidence is equal
   b. False Bleeding into the skin and mucous membranes is typical as with other platelet disorders
   c. False This occurs in only 10 per cent and is slight
   d. False Megakaryocytes are normal or increased. The problem is increased platelet destruction due to circulating antibodies
   e. True As with any marked thrombocytopenia

7. a. False Low iron concentration with low iron binding capacity is usual. Note that in general serum iron measurement can be unreliable, and serum ferritin is a better indicator of iron stores
   b. True Iron overload is a serious complication
   c. True Due to failure of iron utilisation
   d. False
   e. True It falls rapidly with treatment

8. a. True Both normochromic and hypochromic cells are found
   b. True Due to mixed iron and folate/B_{12} deficiency
   c. False
   d. True Liver disease is the other main cause of a dimorphic picture due to gastrointestinal bleeding plus folate deficiency
   e. False

9. **Thrombocytopenia is a recognised feature of—**

   a. von Willebrand's disease
   b. Systemic lupus erythematosus
   c. Henoch–Schönlein purpura
   d. Wiskott–Aldrich syndrome
   e. Chronic heparin therapy

10. **A microcytic blood picture is seen in—**

    a. Beta-thalassaemia minor
    b. Scurvy
    c. Congenital sideroblastic anaemia
    d. Coeliac disease
    e. Pyruvate kinase deficiency

11. **Characteristic features of von Willebrand's disease include—**

    a. Sex-linked inheritance
    b. Disordered platelet aggregation
    c. Prolonged prothrombin time
    d. Correction of bleeding tendency by administration of serum from haemophiliacs
    e. Bleeding into large joints

12. **A patient has a monoclonal paraprotein band on electrophoresis. Indications that it represents malignant disease include—**

    a. Bence-Jones protein in the urine
    b. Erythrocyte sedimentation rate (ESR) greater than 100 mm/h
    c. Depression of other immunoglobulin fractions
    d. Presence of bone lesions
    e. Paraprotein level of 30 g/l

13. **Eosinophilia in the peripheral blood is characteristic of—**

    a. Schistosomiasis
    b. Kala-azar
    c. Rubella
    d. Chronic active hepatitis
    e. Loeffler's syndrome

Answers overleaf

9. a. False   Though platelet function is disturbed
    b. True   Due to antiplatelet antibodies
    c. False
    d. True   A sex-linked syndrome including eczema and depressed immunity
    e. True

10. a. True
    b. False   It is normocytic or occasionally slightly macrocytic
    c. True
    d. True   A macrocytic or dimorphic blood picture may also occur
    e. False

11. a. False   It is usually autosomal dominant, but occasionally autosomal recessive
    b. True
    c. False   The bleeding time is prolonged
    d. True
    e. False   Bleeding into mucous membranes and skin is more usual. Contrast haemophilia

12. a. True
    b. False   Both benign and malignant paraprotein peaks cause a very high sedimentation rate
    c. True
    d. True
    e. True   Very high levels and a rising level of paraprotein point towards malignant disease

13. a. True   As with many other parasitic infestations
    b. False   A leucopenia is usual
    c. False
    d. False
    e. True   Remember polyarteritis nodosa, Hodgkin's disease and allergies as the other main causes of eosinophilia

14. **Spherocytes in the peripheral blood are a feature of—**

    a. Autoimmune haemolytic anaemia
    b. Splenectomy
    c. Multiple myeloma
    d. Severe burns
    e. Lead poisoning

15. **Clinically detectable splenomegaly is characteristic of—**

    a. Hereditary spherocytosis
    b. Sickle cell disease in an adult
    c. Beta-thalassaemia major
    d. Glucose-6-phosphate dehydrogenase deficiency
    e. Autoimmune haemolytic anaemia

16. **A neutrophil leucocytosis is characteristic of—**

    a. Influenza
    b. Leptospirosis
    c. Legionnaire's disease
    d. Typhoid
    e. Pertussis

17. **A 55-year-old man has massive splenomegaly. Features that suggest chronic myeloid leukaemia rather than myelofibrosis include—**

    a. A white cell count greater than $50 \times 10^9/l$ (50 000 per mm^3)
    b. Elevated neutrophil alkaline phosphatase level
    c. Nucleated red blood cells in the peripheral blood
    d. Presence of Philadelphia chromosome
    e. Anaemia

18. **Features of polycythaemia (rubra) vera include—**

    a. Reduced plasma volume
    b. Haemorrhagic tendency
    c. Elevated ESR
    d. Pruritus
    e. Increased neutrophil alkaline phosphatase level

Answers overleaf

14. a. True Hereditary spherocytosis, an intrinsic red cell abnormality, is not the only cause. Spherocytes are produced as a result of extrinsic damage (e.g. autoantibodies, severe burns and infection)

  b. False Howell–Jolly bodies are characteristic
  c. False
  d. True
  e. False

15. a. True
  b. False By adult life the spleen is shrunken from repeated infarction
  c. True
  d. False Splenomegaly is not prominent
  e. True

16. a. False Significant leucocytosis might suggest secondary bacterial infection
  b. True Helpful in distinguishing the causes of hepatitis
  c. True
  d. False Leucopenia is usual. A sudden leucocytosis suggests intestinal perforation
  e. False Lymphocytosis is characteristic

17. a. True The white cell count may be elevated in myelofibrosis but rarely to this degree
  b. False It is low in chronic myeloid. In myelofibrosis it is normal or increased
  c. False Primitive red cells are typical of myelofibrosis
  d. True
  e. False Anaemia occurs in both

18. a. False The plasma volume is normal. The red cell volume is increased and therefore the total blood volume is increased
  b. True Surgery is a particular hazard. Vascular engorgement and platelet abnormalities are two contributory factors to the bleeding tendency
  c. False It is rarely greater than 1 mm in the first hour
  d. True Histamine release is thought to be responsible
  e. True In about 70 per cent of cases

19. Characteristic features of multiple myeloma include—

    a. Generalised lymphadenopathy
    b. Bone pain
    c. Raised alkaline phosphatase
    d. Onset in 30–50 year age group
    e. Hypercalcaemia

20. Bone marrow failure may be a feature of—

    a. Human immunodeficiency virus infection
    b. Miliary tuberculosis
    c. Zieve's syndrome
    d. Paroxysmal nocturnal haemoglobinuria
    e. Cotrimoxazole therapy

21. Features of chronic lymphatic leukaemia include—

    a. Malignant cells generally with T-lymphocyte characteristics
    b. M band on plasma protein electrophoresis of serum
    c. More common in women than men
    d. Coombs-positive haemolytic anaemia
    e. Hypogammaglobulinaemia

22. In Hodgkin's disease—

    a. Cell-mediated immunity is better preserved than humoral immunity
    b. There is a female preponderance
    c. Eosinophilia is a recognised feature
    d. The presence of constitutional symptoms is a bad prognostic sign
    e. Renal colic is a recognised complication

23. Well-recognised complications of sickle cell disease include—

    a. Proliferative retinopathy
    b. Generalised osteoporosis
    c. Leukaemic transformation
    d. Aseptic necrosis of the hip
    e. Cholelithiasis

Answers overleaf

19. a. False Lymphadenopathy does occur but is quite rare
    b. True
    c. False Usually normal as osteoblastic activity is not increased
    d. False Older
    e. True

20. a. True
    b. True
    c. False Haemolysis in association with hyperlipidaemia in alcoholic hepatitis
    d. True
    e. True Folic acid antagonist

21. a. False Usually B-lymphocyte characteristics
    b. True Small amounts of paraprotein may be detected
    c. False Male to female ratio approximately 2:1
    d. True
    e. True Immune paresis

22. a. False
    b. False Male to female ratio approximately 3:1
    c. True
    d. True
    e. True Increased cell turnover, especially during treatment, may cause hyperuricaemia

23. a. True As a consequence of retinal ischaemia
    b. False Bony infarcts are common and biconcave 'fish mouth' vertebra characteristic
    c. False
    d. True
    e. True It may be difficult to differentiate acute cholecystitis from painful abdominal sickling crises

24. An attack of acute intermittent porphyria is characterised by—

    a. Diarrhoea
    b. Confusion
    c. Hypotension
    d. Bullous rash
    e. Abdominal pain

25. Characteristic features of porphyria cutanea tarda (symptomatic cutaneous hepatic porphyria) include—

    a. An association with alcohol abuse
    b. Neurological symptoms
    c. Need for iron supplements
    d. Photosensitivity
    e. Increased urinary porphobilinogen

Answers overleaf

24. a. False Constipation is usual
     b. True   A variety of psychiatric manifestations are seen
     c. False Hypertension and tachycardia are usual
     d. False Skin problems are not a feature of this type of porphyria
     e. True

25. a. True   Excess alcohol and an enzyme defect are probably the main factors in causation
     b. False Unlike acute intermittent porphyria
     c. False Iron overload is the rule. Venesection is standard treatment
     d. True
     e. False These are hard to remember, but this is the finding in acute intermittent porphyria

Immunology

1. **Circulating immune complexes are important in the pathogenesis of—**

   a. Goodpasture's syndrome
   b. Pernicious anaemia
   c. Nephrotic syndrome due to malaria
   d. Serum sickness
   e. Myasthenia gravis

2. **Disorders that cause depression primarily of the cell-mediated immune system include—**

   a. DiGeorge's syndrome
   b. Hodgkin's disease
   c. Chronic granulomatous disease
   d. Sarcoidosis
   e. Nephrotic syndrome

3. **Chronic granulomatous disease is characterised by—**

   a. Inability of neutrophils to phagocytose bacteria
   b. Chronically enlarged lymph nodes
   c. Recurrent candidiasis
   d. Dominant inheritance
   e. Hypogammaglobulinaemia

4. **IgM—**

   a. Antibodies are responsible for haemolysis in rhesus incompatibility
   b. Is a potent activator of complement
   c. Is the predominant immunoglobulin elevated in chronic active hepatitis
   d. Is the predominant antibody in the secondary response to antigen
   e. Is the predominant immunoglobulin involved in warm type autoimmune haemolytic anaemia

Answers overleaf

1. a. False Antibodies react directly with the glomerular basement membrane, being deposited in a linear fashion, in contrast to the lumpy deposition of immune complex nephritis

  b. False Again autoantibodies bind locally

  c. True A number of other infective agents also act as antigens in immune complex nephritis

  d. True

  e. False

2. a. True There is a failure of thymic development and hence T-lymphocyte deficiency

  b. True Subsequent treatment may affect humoral immunity

  c. False Humoral immunity is depressed due to hypogammaglobulinaemia

  d. True Remember the negative Mantoux test

  e. False Erysipelas and pneumococcal peritonitis were common in the preantibiotic era. Defence against these agents is primarily antibody-mediated

3. a. False The problem is inability to kill ingested bacteria

  b. True They may suppurate, break down and form sinuses

  c. False Bacteria such as staphylococci and gram-negative species predominate

  d. False It is usually X-linked

  e. False Gammaglobulins may be elevated in response to chronic infection

4. a. False IgG is the main immunoglobulin that crosses the placenta

  b. True Due to the many binding sites for antigen
It is IgG

  c. False IgM is the first immunoglobulin produced

  d. False IgM is responsible for the cold type, except

  e. False paroxysmal cold haemoglobinuria

5. Tests directed at assessment of the cell-mediated immune system include—

    a. Skin prick testing
    b. Nitroblue tetrazolium test
    c. Response of lymphocytes to phytohaemagglutinin
    d. Mantoux testing
    e. Patch testing

6. Late onset hypogammaglobulinaemia (common variable immunodeficiency)—

    a. Results in recurrent virus infection of the upper respiratory tract
    b. Is associated with autoimmune disorders
    c. Predisposes to carcinoma of the stomach
    d. Is diagnosed by the absence of B-lymphocytes in the peripheral blood
    e. Is inherited in an X-linked recessive manner

Answers overleaf

5. a. False A test of type I hypersensitivity
   b. False This is a test of polymorphonuclear leucocyte function
   c. True The proliferation of T-lymphocytes in response to this is measured
   d. True This identifies T-lymphocytes
   e. True

6. a. False Bacterial infections are characteristic
   b. True
   c. True Achlorhydria may be relevant
   d. False B-lymphocytes are often present but do not produce antibody
   e. False Not familial

Infectious and Tropical Diseases

1. **Manifestations of *Listeria monocytogenes* infection include—**

   a. Skin rash in veterinary workers
   b. Toxin-mediated diarrhoea
   c. Meningoencephalitis in neonates
   d. Generalised lymphadenopathy
   e. Increased severity of infection during pregnancy

2. **Recognised complications of chickenpox include—**

   a. Pancreatitis
   b. Cerebellar ataxia
   c. Purpura
   d. Viral pneumonia, especially in adults
   e. Hepatitis

3. **Characteristic features of typhoid fever include—**

   a. Polymorph leucocytosis
   b. Watery diarrhoea
   c. Reduced mental alertness
   d. Bullous rash
   e. Splenomegaly

4. ***Cryptococcus neoformans—***

   a. Is a filamentous fungus
   b. Complicates lymphomas
   c. Is characteristically found in soil contaminated by pigeon droppings
   d. Produces symptoms in the respiratory system most commonly
   e. Is resistant to amphotericin B

5. **Recognised presentations of *Taenia solium* infestation include—**

   a. Urticarial rash
   b. Epilepsy
   c. Macrocytic anaemia
   d. Liver abscess
   e. Weight loss

Answers overleaf

1. a. True   Maculopapular eruption on the hands
   b. False   But diarrhoea may occur with heavy infection
   c. True   Also in the elderly and immunocompromised
   d. True
   e. False   During pregnancy there is increased susceptibility to infection which is often less severe

2. a. False   It does complicate certain virus infections, typically mumps
   b. True   Due to encephalitis
   c. True
   d. True   The pneumonia in adults can be serious
   e. True   A rare complication

3. a. False   Leucopenia is characteristic
   b. False   Constipation is usual
   c. True
   d. False   A macular rash is typical
   e. True

4. a. False   It is a yeast and, unlike some other yeasts, cannot change to a mycelium
   b. True   Immunosuppression predisposes to many fungal infections
   c. True   Rich nitrogen content is ideal for fungal survival
   d. False   Neurological symptoms and signs are most common
   e. False   Amphotericin is quite effective

5. a. True   At the stage of cysticercal invasion
   b. True
   c. False   Do not confuse *Diphyllobothrium latum*
   d. False   Do not confuse hydatid disease
   e. True   A symptom of adult worm infestation

6. **Recognised features of *Schistosoma mansoni* infestation include—**

   a. Diagnosis by rectal biopsy
   b. Interstitial pulmonary fibrosis
   c. Immune complex nephrotic syndrome
   d. Splenomegaly
   e. Diarrhoea

7. **Characteristic features of tuberculoid leprosy include—**

   a. Positive lepromin test
   b. Isolation of organisms from the skin
   c. Symmetrical peripheral neuropathy
   d. Negligible risk of person-to-person spread
   e. Iritis

8. **The following infections characteristically have an incubation period of less than 7 days—**

   a. Scarlet fever
   b. Measles
   c. Cholera
   d. Typhoid
   e. Brucellosis

9. **Complications of infectious mononucleosis include—**

   a. Haemolytic anaemia
   b. Meningitis
   c. Facial nerve palsy
   d. Splenic rupture
   e. Hepatitis

10. **Characteristic features of yellow fever include—**

    a. A relative bradycardia accompanying fever
    b. Severe frontal headache
    c. Centrizonal necrosis of the liver
    d. Bleeding tendency
    e. Good response to penicillin

Answers overleaf

6. a. True
    b. True   When eggs bypass the liver via portacaval anastomoses
    c. True
    d. True   Due to portal hypertension
    e. True   Due to bowel involvement

7. a. True   Due to well-developed hypersensitivity
    b. False Unlike lepromatous leprosy
    c. False This is typical of lepromatous leprosy. In tuberculoid leprosy, nerves (e.g. greater auricular) are singled out here and there
    d. True   The risk is greater in lepromatous leprosy
    e. False A feature of lepromatous leprosy

8. a. True   2–5 days
    b. False 7–14 days
    c. True   Usually a few hours
    d. False 7–21 days
    e. False 7–28 days

9. a. True   In general complications are rare but can be dramatic
    b. True
    c. True
    d. True
    e. True   Subclinical hepatitis is common

10. a. True   Faget's sign
    b. True   Common presenting symptom
    c. False Midzonal necrosis, which is also seen in Lassa fever, is characteristic
    d. True
    e. False The cause is a togavirus, which is not penicillin sensitive

11. A bleeding tendency is a recognised feature of—

    a. Leptospirosis
    b. Poliomyelitis
    c. Ebola virus disease
    d. Cholera
    e. Yellow fever

12. There is negligible risk of person-to-person spread of infection in—

    a. Marburg virus disease
    b. Mumps, once salivary gland swelling appears
    c. Brucellosis
    d. Measles, once the rash appears
    e. Varicella, before the rash appears

13. *Clostridium tetani*—

    a. Is a gram-negative bacillus
    b. Forms spores easily
    c. Is microaerophilic
    d. Can be killed effectively by administration of antiserum
    e. Causes most severe illness following a very short incubation period

14. Characteristically the rash of typhoid fever—

    a. Is worse on the face and limbs
    b. Appears in the first few days of the illness
    c. Is due to petechial haemorrhages
    d. Lasts up to 2 weeks
    e. Helps to differentiate typhoid fever from paratyphoid fever

15. Recognised features of congenital cytomegalovirus infection include—

    a. Markedly increased incidence of congenital heart defects
    b. Chorioretinitis
    c. Purpura
    d. Recurrent respiratory infection
    e. Hepatosplenomegaly

Answers overleaf

11.   a.   True   Due to liver disease
      b.   False
      c.   True   Probably due to disseminated intravascular coagulation
      d.   False
      e.   True

12.   a.   False   Contact with blood, urine and semen of infected cases causes the disease
      b.   False   Although the maximal infectivity is before swelling occurs
      c.   True   Person-to-person spread is very rare
      d.   False   Infectivity persists for about another 4 days
      e.   False   It is infectious for about 5 days before

13.   a.   False   It is gram-positive
      b.   True   Hence its ability to survive
      c.   False   A strict anaerobe
      d.   False   Antiserum neutralises the toxin
      e.   True

14.   a.   False   Worse on the trunk
      b.   False   Second week
      c.   False   Macules which fade on pressure
      d.   False   Usually disappears in 2–3 days
      e.   False   A similar rash occurs in both diseases

15.   a.   False   Unlike congenital rubella
      b.   True
      c.   True
      d.   True
      e.   True   Other features include microcephaly, deafness and cerebral calcification

16. Brucellosis—

    a. Results from infection with gram-negative rods
    b. Produces IgM agglutinating antibodies, which persist long after clinical recovery
    c. Is best treated with benzylpenicillin
    d. Is a cause of spondylitis
    e. Is characterised by a relative lymphocytosis

17. Characteristic features of diphtheria include—

    a. Incubation period of less than 7 days
    b. Spread by droplet infection
    c. Little benefit from the administration of antitoxin
    d. Most marked toxin formation when primary infection is in the nose
    e. Bulbar palsy

18. Features more typical of *Shigella* dysentery than typhoid include—

    a. Chronic carrier state
    b. Osteomyelitis
    c. Diagnosis by blood culture
    d. Bloody diarrhoea
    e. Leucocytosis

19. In a patient with meningitis particular suspicion that the organism is a pneumococcus is raised if there is a history of—

    a. Feeling poorly with headaches for some weeks
    b. Chronic ear infection
    c. Sudden onset of the illness in a fit, young army recruit
    d. Ventriculovenous shunt for control of hydrocephalus
    e. Previous splenectomy

Answers overleaf

16. a. True
    b. True   Thus difficulty may arise in differentiating those with acute illness from those with previous exposure. IgG antibodies tend to disappear with resolution of clinical illness
    c. False   Tetracyclines are the usual choice
    d. True
    e. True   The total white cell count is normal or slightly reduced

17. a. True
    b. True
    c. False   Since its use mortality has fallen dramatically
    d. False   Oropharyngeal involvement is associated with maximum toxin formation
    e. True

18. a. False   Carriage of *Shigella* is rare. Numerous infamous typhoid carriers are well documented
    b. False   May complicate typhoid
    c. False   Septicaemia is rare with *Shigella*
    d. True   In typhoid constipation is usual although diarrhoea may occur
    e. True   Slight leucocytosis is common, while in typhoid leucopenia is usual

19. a. False   Typical of tuberculous meningitis
    b. True
    c. False   This would be typical of meningococcal meningitis
    d. False   *Staphylococcus albus* is a particularly common cause of meningitis in these patients, although it is normally a skin commensal
    e. True   Particularly in younger patients, the incidence of infection is increased after splenectomy. The pneumococcus is one of the organisms most commonly involved

20. The human immunodeficiency virus (HIV)—

a. Has a gene that inhibits reverse transcriptase
b. Shows characteristic trophism for helper T-cells
c. Is easily destroyed by formalin
d. Produces a brief antibody response which is not usually detectable during clinical illness
e. Is most easily isolated from faeces in infected cases

21. Malignant lesions strongly associated with virus infections include—

a. Hepatocellular carcinoma
b. Carcinoma of the cervix
c. Nasopharyngeal cancer
d. Renal cell carcinoma
e. Chronic lymphatic leukaemia

22. Recognised complications of rubella include—

a. Thrombocytopenia
b. Otitis media
c. Encephalitis
d. Glomerulonephritis
e. Arthritis

23. *Actinomyces*—

a. Is visible under the light microscope as gram-positive branching hyphae
b. Is a common commensal in the mouth
c. Grows within tissues as visible, tight-knit clusters
d. Is usually sensitive to penicillin
e. Grows best in an atmosphere enriched in oxygen

Answers overleaf

20. a. False Reverse transcriptase incorporates the virus into host cell genome
   b. True Numbers of these cells may be reduced
   c. True
   d. False The HIV antibody test is usually positive in patients with clinical illness
   e. False The virus is most easily isolated from semen, blood or saliva

21. a. True Hepatitis B
   b. True
   c. True Epstein–Barr virus
   d. False
   e. False

22. a. True
   b. False
   c. True Rare
   d. False
   e. True Relatively common

23. a. True
   b. True
   c. True So-called 'sulphur' granules
   d. True Prolonged treatment is usually necessary
   e. False It is anaerobic

24. *Neisseria* **meningitis—**

   a. Is gram-positive

   b. Can be found inside polymorphs in the cerebrospinal fluid in patients with meningitis

   c. May produce chronic infection lasting some months, characterised by rashes and arthralgia

   d. Is spread mainly by asymptomatic nasopharyngeal carriers

   e. Produces endotoxin

25. **Granuloma inguinale—**

   a. Is caused by a spirochaete

   b. Is highly infectious

   c. Presents with a painful nodule

   d. Commonly spreads to regional lymph nodes

   e. Responds well to tetracyclines

Answers overleaf

24. a. False   Gram-negative cocci
    b. True   The intracellular location is typical
    c. True   Such chronic meningococcaemia is uncommon
    d. True   Only small numbers in the population will get the disease, but 5–10 per cent are carriers
    e. True   Causes circulatory collapse in severe infection

25. a. False   Coccobacillus, *Calymmatobacterium granulomatis*
    b. False
    c. False   Usually painless
    d. False   Unlike lymphogranuloma venereum and chancroid
    e. True

Neurology

1. **Recognised features of lesions in the frontal lobe include—**

   a. Astereognosis
   b. Positive grasp reflex
   c. Superior homonymous quadrantanopia
   d. Unilateral optic atrophy
   e. Anosmia

2. **Features of syringobulbia include—**

   a. Rotatory nystagmus
   b. Optic atrophy
   c. Weakness of sternomastoid
   d. High cerebrospinal fluid protein levels
   e. Vocal cord paralysis

3. **Calcification on skull X-ray is found in—**

   a. Vitamin B_{12} deficiency
   b. Sturge–Weber syndrome
   c. Hypoparathyroidism
   d. Cushing's disease
   e. Chronic subdural haematoma

4. **In Parkinson's disease—**

   a. Blepharospasm is a recognised feature
   b. Somnolence suggests a postencephalitic aetiology
   c. Tendon reflexes are normal
   d. Dyskinesia is a complication of treatment with amantadine
   e. Tricyclic antidepressants are contraindicated

5. **Characteristic features of myotonia congenita include—**

   a. Worsening with exposure to heat
   b. Improvement after repeated voluntary activity
   c. Persistence after curarisation
   d. Fasciculation in the affected muscle
   e. Involvement of the long flexors of the hands

Answers overleaf

1. a. False   This is characteristic of parietal lobe lesions
    b. True
    c. False   This is a feature of temporal lobe lesions
    d. True   This may be produced by pressure on the optic nerve. Associated with increased intracranial pressure papilloedema may occur in the other eye (Foster Kennedy syndrome)
    e. True   The olfactory nerve lies beneath the frontal lobe

2. a. True
    b. False
    c. True   Involvement of the accessory nerve
    d. False
    e. True   Involvement of the 10th cranial nerve nucleus

3. a. False
    b. True   Later in life
    c. True   Calcification in the basal ganglia is found in about half these patients
    d. False
    e. True

4. a. True   Also blepharoclonus
    b. False   This is characteristic of the precipitating illness—encephalitis lethargica
    c. True
    d. False   May be an unwanted effect of treatment with levodopa
    e. False   Depression is common in Parkinson's disease

5. a. False   Cold usually exacerbates
    b. True
    c. True   The defect is in the muscle membrane
    d. False
    e. True   It is a generalised condition, although the tongue is also very characteristically affected

6. **Characteristic features of motor neurone disease include—**

   a. Fasciculation
   b. Retention of urine
   c. Early loss of abdominal reflexes
   d. Nystagmus
   e. Intellectual deterioration

7. **Transient monocular visual loss is a recognised feature of—**

   a. Internal carotid artery occlusion
   b. Occipital lobe infarction
   c. Retinal detachment
   d. Motor neurone disease
   e. Disseminated sclerosis

8. **A prolapsed intervertebral disc between L4 and L5 vertebrae can produce on the affected side—**

   a. An absent knee jerk
   b. Impaired dorsiflexion of the foot
   c. Reduced sensation over the great toe
   d. An absent ankle jerk
   e. Reduced straight leg raising

9. **Characteristic causes of a predominantly motor peripheral neuropathy include—**

   a. Acute intermittent porphyria
   b. Diphtheria
   c. B_{12} deficiency
   d. Leprosy
   e. Guillain–Barré syndrome

10. **Ptosis is a recognised feature of—**

   a. Friedreich's ataxia
   b. Wilson's disease
   c. Dystrophia myotonica
   d. Occlusion of the posterior inferior cerebellar artery
   e. Facial nerve palsy

Answers overleaf

6. a. True   Fasciculation occurs in lower motor neurone lesions, especially when damage is near the anterior horn cell

    b. False   Urinary problems are unusual and occur late in the disease

    c. False   These may be preserved until late, unlike multiple sclerosis where they are lost early

    d. False   Oddly the ocular nuclei are rarely affected

    e. False   The intellect may be intact to the end

7. a. True

    b. False   Hemianopia with macular sparing

    c. True

    d. False

    e. True   Typically, visual loss improves over 2–3 weeks

8. a. False   Between L4 and L5 vertebrae the affected nerve root is L5. The knee jerk is controlled by roots L3 and L4

    b. True   This movement is controlled by roots L4 and L5

    c. True

    d. False   The ankle jerk is controlled by S1 and S2 roots

    e. True

9. a. True

    b. True   Remember the respiratory paralysis

    c. False   There are prominent sensory findings as well

    d. False

    e. True   The other predominant motor neuropathy is lead poisoning

10. a. False

    b. False

    c. True

    d. True   Due to interruption of the sympathetic supply in the lateral medulla

    e. False

11. **In the treatment of acute bacterial meningitis in adults—**

    a. Due to *Haemophilus influenzae* intrathecal antibiotics are indicated
    b. Concurrent administration of intrathecal corticosteroids improves prognosis
    c. A mortality of under 5 per cent is usual
    d. Prophylactic anticonvulsants are indicated
    e. Due to meningococcus, benzylpenicillin is the first-line treatment

12. **Characteristic features of temporal lobe epilepsy include—**

    a. *Jamais vu* experiences
    b. A better response to drug therapy than with other types of epilepsy
    c. Olfactory hallucinations
    d. Outbursts of antisocial behaviour
    e. Total recall of seizure

13. **Causes of cerebellar ataxia include—**

    a. Motor neurone disease
    b. Chronic alcoholism
    c. Phenytoin
    d. Vitamin B_{12} deficiency
    e. Bronchial carcinoma

14. **Cauda equina lesions characteristically produce—**

    a. Hyperreflexia of the lower limbs
    b. Impotence
    c. Loss of abdominal reflexes
    d. Sensory loss over saddle area of the buttocks
    e. Loss of tone of the anal sphincter

15. **Characteristic features of a lesion in the lateral part of the medulla include—**

    a. Ipsilateral Horner's syndrome
    b. Contralateral loss of proprioception to the body and limbs
    c. Nystagmus
    d. Ipsilateral palsy of the hypoglossal nerve
    e. Dysphagia

Answers overleaf

11. a. False
    b. False   Benefit from systemic steroids in children is controversial
    c. False   Considerably higher
    d. False
    e. True

12. a. True   More common than *déjà vu*
    b. False   Good control of seizures is often difficult
    c. True   As well as other types of hallucination
    d. True
    e. False   Amnesia for part or all of the event is common

13. a. False
    b. True   As part of Wernicke's encephalopathy
    c. True
    d. False   Ataxia due to peripheral sensory loss may be present
    e. True   Due either to secondary deposits or a non-metastatic effect

14. a. False   The cauda equina contains lower motor neurones
    b. True
    c. False   This would reflect an upper motor neurone lesion
    d. True   The area supplied by the sacral nerve roots
    e. True

15. a. True
    b. False   The medial lemniscus carrying proprioception is sited medially in the medulla
    c. True
    d. False   The 12th nerve nucleus is sited medially
    e. True   Due to involvement of the 9th and 10th nerves

16. **Characteristic features of infective polyneuritis (Guillain–Barré syndrome) include—**

    a. Pathological changes in the distal parts of the peripheral nerve
    b. Incontinence
    c. Sparing of cranial nerves
    d. Marked improvement with ACTH
    e. High pyrexia

17. **Recognised features of myasthenia gravis include—**

    a. Asymmetrical weakness
    b. An association with systemic lupus erythematosus
    c. Dysphagia
    d. Absent reflexes
    e. Natural remission

18. **In facioscapulohumeral muscular dystrophy—**

    a. Inheritance is autosomal dominant
    b. The patient usually needs a wheelchair by age 20 years
    c. Tendon reflexes are lost early
    d. Creatine kinase levels may be normal
    e. Winging of the scapulae is characteristic

19. **Characteristic findings in the cerebrospinal fluid of a patient with multiple sclerosis include—**

    a. Positive syphilitic serology
    b. Oligoclonal pattern of immunoglobulins on electrophoresis
    c. Total protein of 1.2 g/l (120 mg/100 ml)
    d. Increased white cell count, especially polymorphs
    e. Normal globulin/albumin ratio

20. **Cerebrospinal fluid with increased protein and reduced glucose is seen in—**

    a. Sarcoidosis of the central nervous system
    b. Echovirus meningitis
    c. Meningeal carcinomatosis
    d. Tuberculous meningitis
    e. Leptospirosis

Answers overleaf

16. a. False It is primarily a radiculopathy with changes in the nerve root
    b. False
    c. False They are commonly involved
    d. False The effect is debatable
    e. False Low-grade pyrexia is usual

17. a. True Some groups of muscles (e.g. extraocular) may be profoundly affected, while others are spared
    b. True It is also associated with other autoimmune diseases
    c. True
    d. False Generally reflexes and muscle bulk are preserved, except perhaps in very longstanding cases
    e. True Most remissions and most deaths occur in the first few years after the onset

18. a. True
    b. False The course is often quite benign
    c. False Reflexes are often spared until late in myopathies
    d. True Reflecting the less florid process
    e. True

19. a. False
    b. True
    c. False Some increase in protein is usual but not to this degree
    d. False Increased lymphocytes may be seen
    e. False Usually abnormal and a valuable diagnostic test

20. a. True
    b. False A few causes of viral meningitis may cause a reduction in glucose (e.g. mumps)
    c. True
    d. True At first the glucose level may be normal, but if the lumbar puncture is repeated later, glucose is usually low
    e. True

21. Characteristic clinical features of multiple sclerosis include—

a. Spastic bladder
b. Hearing loss
c. Nystagmus
d. Homonymous hemianopia
e. Aphasia

22. High serum creatine kinase concentrations are commonly found in muscle disease due to—

a. Hypothyroidism
b. Clofibrate
c. Polymyositis
d. Cushing's syndrome
e. Myotonia dystrophica

23. Findings in tabes dorsalis include—

a. Generalised hypertonia
b. Bilateral ptosis
c. Pupils that react to light but not to accommodation
d. Extensor plantars
e. Trophic ulcers

24. Characteristic features of a migraine attack include—

a. Neck stiffness
b. Facial flushing
c. Relief with pizotifen
d. Association with focal epilepsy
e. Total blindness

25. Fasciculation is a feature of—

a. Friedreich's ataxia
b. Poliomyelitis
c. Syringobulbia
d. Myotonia dystrophica
e. Parkinson's disease

Answers overleaf

21. a. True
  b. False Although almost any neurological lesion may occur, certain features are unusual. Hearing loss is extremely uncommon
  c. True Caused by damage to the medial longitudinal fasciculus
  d. False Hemianopias are rare
  e. False Again rare

22. a. True
  b. True
  c. True But not always
  d. False
  e. True Mild to moderate elevation is common

23. a. False Hypotonia is typical
  b. True
  c. False The reverse is true
  d. False Tabes affects primarily the dorsal columns, not upper motor neurones
  e. True

24. a. False
  b. True
  c. False This agent is of value in prophylaxis of attacks
  d. False This would suggest a structural lesion
  e. False Very rare. Visual scintillations, photophobia, etc. are common

25. a. False
  b. True Typical of anterior horn cell lesions
  c. True Of the tongue due to involvement of the hypo-glossal nerve
  d. False
  e. False

Occupational Diseases

1. **In decompression sickness—**
   a. Pruritus is a characteristic symptom
   b. Paraplegia complicates severe cases
   c. Treatment is by prompt recompression
   d. Symptoms of the 'bends' take about 6 hours to develop
   e. Haematocrit usually falls

2. **Characteristic features of poisoning with tetraethyl lead include—**
   a. Colic
   b. Raised total blood lead concentration
   c. Mental confusion
   d. Severe anaemia
   e. Rapid response of symptoms to ethylenediaminetetra-acetic acid (EDTA)

3. **There is a recognised risk of lung cancer associated with exposure to—**
   a. Tin
   b. Chromium
   c. Nickel
   d. Aluminium
   e. Uranium

4. **Characteristic features of chronic cadmium poisoning include—**
   a. Peripheral neuropathy
   b. Proteinuria
   c. Anosmia
   d. Emphysema
   e. Confusion

5. **Industrial injuries benefit under the Prescribed Diseases regulations may be claimed by—**
   a. A farmworker with brucellosis
   b. An aniline dye worker with gastric ulcer
   c. A nurse with tuberculosis
   d. A flax worker with byssinosis
   e. A docker with a prolapsed intervertebral disc

Answers overleaf

1. a. True
   b. True
   c. True
   d. False   Usually they occur within the hour. The 'chokes' may take some hours to appear
   e. False   Haematocrit is often elevated

2. a. False   The point is that the features of organic and inorganic lead poisoning are quite different. Colic is more typical of inorganic poisoning
   b. False   Best detected by urinary lead estimation
   c. True   This dominates the pictures. Acute mania is seen
   d. False   Mild anaemia is a feature of inorganic lead poisoning
   e. False   EDTA cannot bind triethyl lead, the prevalent metabolite of tetraethyl lead

3. a. False   Tin may give X-ray abnormalities, but appears to be harmless
   b. True   Cancer of the nose also occurs
   c. True
   d. False   Fumes produce an acute respiratory disorder which is occasionally complicated by pneumothorax
   e. True

4. a. False
   b. True   The lesion is in the renal tubules
   c. True   With atrophy of the nasal mucosa
   d. True
   e. False

5. a. True   To apply, the disease must be one that is listed, and the occupation one where exposure to the risk has occurred
   b. False   There is no association
   c. True
   d. True
   e. False   Although a docker might acquire such a lesion in his work, a prolapsed disc is not a Prescribed Disease

6. Characteristic features of byssinosis include—

a. Increase in symptoms as the working week progresses
b. Bilateral basal inspiratory crepitations
c. Finger clubbing
d. Patchy infiltrates on chest radiograph
e. Resistance to standard bronchodilator medications

Answers overleaf

6. a. False Exacerbations on return to work, e.g. Monday, are characteristic
   b. False Airways narrowing and rhonchi are typical
   c. False
   d. False Chest radiograph is either normal or shows changes in keeping with chronic bronchitis
   e. False Bronchodilators may be quite helpful

Ophthalmology

1. **Causes of optic atrophy include—**

   a. Syphilis
   b. Motor neurone disease
   c. Friedreich's ataxia
   d. Isoniazid
   e. Malnutrition

2. **Causes of papilloedema include—**

   a. Benign intracranial hypertension
   b. Normal pressure hydrocephalus
   c. Hypocalcaemia
   d. Carbon monoxide poisoning
   e. Hypercapnia

3. **Pupillary dilatation is a recognised feature of—**

   a. Holmes–Adie syndrome
   b. Third nerve palsy
   c. Wernicke's encephalopathy
   d. Poisoning with tricyclic antidepressants
   e. Motor neurone disease

4. **Anterior uveitis is a characteristic feature of—**

   a. Rheumatoid arthritis
   b. Sarcoidosis
   c. Thyrotoxicosis
   d. Reiter's syndrome
   e. Hypoparathyroidism

5. **Dry eyes are a recognised feature of—**

   a. Ankylosing spondylitis
   b. Riley–Day syndrome
   c. Sarcoidosis
   d. Seventh nerve palsy
   e. Horner's syndrome

Answers overleaf

1. a. True   A classic finding in tabes, but also a feature of general paresis
   b. False   The optic nerve is a sensory nerve
   c. True   But is quite uncommon
   d. True   We tend to remember the periperal neuropathy, but optic atrophy also occurs. Ethambutol also causes optic atrophy
   e. True

2. a. True
   b. False
   c. False   Hypercalcaemia is an unusual cause
   d. True
   e. True

3. a. True   Occasionally; but the characteristic feature is its slow reaction to light
   b. True   Due to removal of the parasympathetic supply
   c. False
   d. True   Due to anticholinergic properties
   e. False   Oddly the ocular nuclei (3rd, 4th and 6th cranial nerves) are spared, so pupils and eye movements are normal

4. a. False   It is not characteristic. Scleritis is the typical finding
   b. True
   c. False
   d. True   As with other causes of seronegative arthritis
   e. False   Cataract is the usual ophthalmic problem

5. a. False   Dry eyes occur in Sjögren's syndrome which is usually associated with seropositive arthritis
   b. True   In this inherited disease the autonomic nervous system is disturbed and dry eyes are just one of many consequences
   c. True   Uveitis is characteristic but involvement of the lacrimal glands may cause dry eyes
   d. True   Failure of lid closure allows drying
   e. False

6. Retinal exudates are a characteristic finding in—

    a. Marfan's syndrome
    b. Tabes dorsalis
    c. Retinal vein thrombosis
    d. Amyloidosis
    e. Gaucher's disease

Answers overleaf

6. a. False Lens dislocation is characteristic
   b. False Optic atrophy may occur
   c. True
   d. False
   e. False Cherry-red macular spots are a feature of some of the other lipid storage diseases

Paediatrics

1. **Characteristic features of Fallot's tetralogy include—**

   a. Right axis shift on ECG
   b. Plethoric lung fields
   c. Loud pulmonary second sound
   d. Palliation by anastomosing the left subclavian artery to the pulmonary artery
   e. Cyanosis at birth

2. **Findings recognised as having no pathological significance in a 5-year-old include the presence of—**

   a. Fixed splitting of the second heart sound
   b. A third heart sound
   c. A sound heard in the upper chest, in systole and diastole, which disappears when the neck veins are occluded
   d. Pansystolic murmur
   e. Ejection click

3. **In a neonate an unconjugated bilirubin concentration of 200 mmol/l with little or no rise in the conjugated bilirubin level is recognised in—**

   a. Rhesus incompatibility
   b. Dubin–Johnson syndrome
   c. Neonatal hepatitis
   d. Glucose-6-phosphate dehydrogenase deficiency
   e. Premature delivery

4. **Characteristically a child of 9 months should be able to—**

   a. Grasp an object between finger and thumb
   b. Drink from a cup unaided
   c. Stand while holding on to support
   d. Comprehend simple commands
   e. Use 6–10 recognisable words

Answers overleaf

1. a. True   Left axis shift in a child with cyanotic congenital heart disease raises the possibility of tricuspid atresia
    b. False   Flow to the pulmonary arteries is reduced by right ventricular outflow obstruction
    c. False   It is soft or inaudible
    d. True   This is Blalock-Taussig's operation. Definitive repair is done earlier now and palliative operations are less often required
    e. False   Characteristically develops after the first few weeks of life

2. a. False   This is the typical finding with atrial septal defects
    b. True   This is recognised as physiological until the age of 30 years
    c. True   These features are characteristic of a venous hum
    d. False
    e. False

3. a. True   Due to haemolysis
    b. False   The main defect in Dubin–Johnson syndrome is in excretion of conjugated bilirubin from the liver cell
    c. False   Again the main increase is in conjugated bilirubin
    d. True   Due to haemolysis
    e. True   Various mechanisms including immaturity of liver enzymes are responsible

4. a. True   In a scissor fashion initially
    b. False   Competence using a cup is acquired at about 18 months
    c. True
    d. False   Response to commands is acquired by 12 months
    e. False   Deliberate vocalisation is only beginning at this stage

5. **Delayed bone age compared to chronological age is a feature of—**

    a. Hypothyroidism
    b. Social deprivation
    c. Congenital adrenal hyperplasia
    d. Constitutional growth delay
    e. Growth hormone excess

6. **Characteristic non-articular features of the systemic variant of Still's disease include—**

    a. Conjunctivitis
    b. Fleeting rash
    c. Leucocytosis
    d. Splenomegaly
    e. Rheumatoid nodules

7. **Characteristic features of acute lymphoblastic leukaemia include—**

    a. Tumour cells which react with anti-B cell monoclonal antibodies
    b. Better prognosis when the white cell count at presentation is very high
    c. Massive splenomegaly
    d. Disseminated intravascular coagulation
    e. Spread to the meninges unless prophylactic treatment to the central nervous system is given

8. **Characteristic features of phenylketonuria include—**

    a. Normal on physical examination at birth
    b. Eczema
    c. Tendency to venous thrombosis
    d. Cataracts
    e. Fair hair

Answers overleaf

5. a. True It is characteristically retarded
   b. True
   c. False Bone age is advanced
   d. True Bone age will be close to height age
   e. False

6. a. False Iridocyclitis is characteristic
   b. True The rash may come and go within hours
   c. True Occasionally a leukemoid reaction is seen
   d. True
   e. False Overall only about 10 per cent have a positive rheumatoid factor and are likely to have nodules. These cases are mostly the subgroup where the disease starts at an older age

7. a. False Cells are usually of the null type
   b. False Although the initial response may be good, ultimately this group will have a poorer prognosis
   c. False Splenomegaly is mild to moderate in acute leukaemias
   d. False This is particularly associated with acute promyelocytic leukaemia
   e. True Before such prophylactic treatment, meningeal involvement often occurred even when otherwise the patient appeared to be in remission

8. a. True Hence the value of biochemical screening
   b. True Perhaps related to phenylalanine restriction
   c. False This is a feature of homocystinuria
   d. False
   e. True

9. **Characteristic features of Henoch–Schönlein purpura include—**

    a. Arthritis
    b. Membranous glomerulonephritis
    c. Rash involving the face
    d. Reduced serum complement
    e. Prolonged bleeding time

10. **Transplacental transfer of blood constituents may cause neonatal disease, when the mother is suffering from—**

    a. Hyperparathyroidism
    b. Guillain–Barré syndrome
    c. Idiopathic thrombocytopenic purpura
    d. Graves' disease
    e. Biliary cirrhosis

11. **Causes of liver cirrhosis in childhood include—**

    a. Galactosaemia
    b. Coeliac disease
    c. Phenylketonuria
    d. Infectious mononucleosis
    e. Wilson's disease

12. **In a boy of 4 years with congenital adrenal hyperplasia—**

    a. The testes are enlarged
    b. Plasma ACTH levels are low
    c. Height is above normal
    d. Adrenalectomy is the treatment of choice
    e. A deficiency of 21-hydroxylase is most often the cause

13. **An infant is born at full term but weighs less than 2.5 kg. Complications that are characteristically associated include—**

    a. Meconium aspiration syndrome
    b. Intraventricular haemorrhage
    c. Hypoglycaemia
    d. Poor feeding
    e. Pulmonary haemorrhage

Answers overleaf

9. a. True
 b. False The glomerulonephritis is usually focal
 c. False Buttocks and extensor surface are most commonly involved. The face can be involved in infants
 d. False
 e. False The platelet count is normal

10. a. True Transient hypocalcaemia may result
 b. False
 c. True Antiplatelet antibodies pass across the placenta
 d. True Transfer of thyroid stimulating immunoglobulin
 e. False

11. a. True It also causes neonatal hepatitis
 b. False
 c. False Though other disturbances of amino acid handling may cause cirrhosis, e.g. tryosinosis, cystinosis
 d. False Hepatitis may occur
 e. True All cases of cirrhosis in childhood should be screened for this

12. a. False They will be small. The excessive androgen comes from the adrenal, and testicular androgen production is suppressed
 b. False They are increased due to the feedback resulting from the enzyme block
 c. True Though dwarfism will ultimately occur because the epiphyses fuse early
 d. False Cortisone is used to suppress the ACTH drive which causes the excessive androgen production
 e. True

13. a. True
 b. False Certain complications tend to be common in the premature (as opposed to small-for-dates) infant and intraventricular haemorrhage is an example
 c. True
 d. False These infants usually feed greedily unless other complications prevent them
 e. True Particularly in association with hypothermia

14. **Muscular hypotonia without significant weakness is a characteristic feature of—**

    a. Cerebral palsy
    b. Prader–Willi syndrome
    c. Down's syndrome
    d. Werdnig–Hoffman disease (spinal muscular atrophy)
    e. Guillain—Barré syndrome

15. **Failure of the anterior fontanelle to close by 18 months is a feature of—**

    a. Rickets
    b. Phenylketonuria
    c. Hydrocephalus
    d. Hypothyroidism
    e. Down's syndrome

16. **Characteristic features of acute bronchiolitis in children include—**

    a. Respiratory syncytial virus is the most common cause
    b. Sporadic rather than epidemic pattern of infection
    c. Marked hyperinflation of lungs on chest radiograph
    d. Good response to early treatment with corticosteroids
    e. Increased risk of apnoeic attacks

17. **Characteristic features of Kawasaki disease include—**

    a. Strawberry tongue
    b. Sudden onset of cardiac failure in a previously well child
    c. Tender lymphadenopathy
    d. Coronary artery aneurysms in fatal cases
    e. Improvement in response to acyclovir

18. **It is generally considered inappropriate to employ immunisation against—**

    a. Pertussis in a child with cerebral palsy
    b. Pneumococcus in chronic sickle cell disease
    c. Measles during a measles epidemic
    d. Tuberculosis in HIV-positive patients
    e. Diphtheria and tetanus before 4 months of age

Answers overleaf

14. a. False Spasticity is usual. Hypotonia is also seen, but would be associated with weakness
    b. True
    c. True
    d. False Weakness is prominent
    e. False

15. a. True
    b. False
    c. True The fontanelle becomes greatly enlarged and tense
    d. True Bone age is generally retarded
    e. False

16. a. True
    b. False Winter epidemics are typical
    c. True
    d. False
    e. True

17. a. True Skin and mucous membrane changes are characteristic
    b. False Cardiac complications usually present in the convalescent phase
    c. True
    d. True
    e. False Is a vasculitis

18. a. False
    b. False Hyposplenism increases risk of pneumococcal infection
    c. False
    d. True Most other live vaccines and inactivated vaccines can be used
    e. False Triple vaccine is now recommended at 2 months

19. Autosomal recessive inheritance is found in—

   a. Hunter's syndrome
   b. Galactosaemia
   c. von Gierke's disease
   d. Tuberous sclerosis
   e. Christmas disease

20. In sex-linked recessive disorders—

   a. Clinical manifestations are usually present at birth
   b. All the sisters of an affected male are usually carriers
   c. Approximately half the brothers of carrier females will have the disease
   d. The parents of an affected male are usually outwardly normal
   e. Half the sons of affected males will have the disease

Answers overleaf

19. a. False It is sex-linked, unlike the other mucopoly-saccharidoses which have autosomal recessive inheritance

     b. True Most of the disorders involving enzyme defects have autosomal recessive inheritance. In this case it is galactose-1-phosphate uridyl transferase

     c. True Glucose-6-phosphatase is deficient

     d. False Autosomal dominant

     e. False Sex-linked recessive

20. a. False In many of these conditions clinical manifestations are delayed

     b. False About half his sisters will be carriers

     c. True Though some female carriers could have new mutations (but to answer 'false' on this basis would be complicating the issue too much)

     d. True

     e. False None will have it

Pharmacology

1. A fixed drug eruption is a characteristic unwanted effect of—

    a. Quinine
    b. Ampicillin
    c. Dapsone
    d. Phenobarbitone
    e. Chlorpromazine

2. Advantages of ACTH over prednisone include a lower incidence of—

    a. Osteoporosis
    b. Fluid retention
    c. Acne
    d. Adrenal insufficiency with intercurrent stress
    e. Growth retardation in children

3. In the treatment of acute intermittent porphyria, drugs that may be safely used include—

    a. Methyldopa for hypertension
    b. Diazepam for sedation
    c. Phenytoin for control of fits
    d. Pethidine for pain relief
    e. Sulphonamide for coincidental infection

4. Photosensitivity is a characteristic unwanted effect of—

    a. Tetracyclines
    b. Propranolol
    c. Sulphonamide
    d. Clonidine
    e. Chlorothiazide

5. Drugs that are metabolized by acetylation in the liver include—

    a. Phenytoin
    b. Hydrallazine
    c. Dapsone
    d. Tolbutamide
    e. Isoniazid

Answers overleaf

1. a. True A fixed eruption is one that recurs at the same site with repeated exposure
  b. False
  c. True
  d. True Sulphonamides are the other common cause
  e. False Photosensitivity is characteristic

2. a. True ACTH causes release of anabolic as well as catabolic steroids
  b. False
  c. False ACTH causes androgen release
  d. True The adrenals are not suppressed as is the case with prednisone
  e. True Again because ACTH has less catabolic effect

3. a. False Methyldopa may precipitate an attack. Propranolol is a better choice
  b. True
  c. False Many antiepileptics including barbiturates and other hydantoins precipitate intermittent porphyria
  d. True Morphine should be avoided
  e. False

4. a. True One of the most common drug causes
  b. False
  c. True
  d. False
  e. True Nalidixic acid and griseofulvin are other causes

5. a. False It is hydroxylated in the liver
  b. True Slow acetylators are more likely to get lupus erythematosus
  c. True
  d. False It is oxidised in the liver
  e. True Slow acetylators are more likely to get peripheral neuropathy

6. Drugs that characteristically cause skin pigmentation as an unwanted effect include—

a. Chlorpromazine
b. Ranitidine
c. Chloroquine
d. Streptomycin
e. Busulphan

7. Pulmonary fibrosis is a recognised unwanted effect of—

a. Amiodarone
b. Bleomycin
c. Colchicine
d. Phenytoin
e. Nitrofurantoin

8. Decreased efficiency of the contraceptive pill is recognised with the use of—

a. Rifampicin
b. Warfarin
c. Phenytoin
d. Cimetidine
e. Hydrallazine

9. Glomerular damage is characteristic of the renal toxicity due to—

a. Penicillamine
b. Gentamicin
c. Naproxen
d. Captopril
e. Amphotericin B

10. Drugs that for the most part are excreted unchanged in the urine include—

a. Gentamicin
b. Isoniazid
c. Rifampicin
d. Chloramphenicol
e. Benzylpenicillin

Answers overleaf

6. a. True
    b. False
    c. True   Pigmentation is common. Pigmentation of the nail beds, bleaching of the hair and retinal changes are also seen
    d. False
    e. True   Pigmentation associated with weakness may simulate Addison's disease

7. a. True
    b. True   As with some other cytotoxic agents, e.g. busulphan
    c. False
    d. False   It may cause hilar lymphadenopathy
    e. True

8. a. True   Due to hepatic enzyme induction
    b. False   However, increased warfarin may be required for adequate anticoagulation
    c. True   The effect, which is also noted with phenobarbitone, is probably due to enzyme induction
    d. False   An enzyme inhibitor
    e. False   Though perhaps a hypertensive patient should not be taking the pill

9. a. True
    b. False   Renal tubular damage is typical
    c. False   Tubular necrosis and interstitial nephritis are the usual lesions
    d. True
    e. False

10. a. True
    b. False   It is acetylated in the liver
    c. False   It is metabolized in the liver
    d. False   It is conjugated to the glucuronide in the liver
    e. True

11. A predominantly cholestatic jaundice may complicate the use of—

    a. Paracetamol
    b. Methyltestosterone
    c. Methyldopa
    d. Chlorpropamide
    e. Primaquine

12. Heparin—

    a. Is a protein
    b. Is contained in mast cells
    c. Has a plasma half-life of about 8 hours
    d. Is secreted in breast milk during therapy
    e. Causes thrombocytopenia

13. Disopyramide—

    a. Has a positive inotropic effect on the heart
    b. Should not be given if the patient is already on digoxin
    c. Is effective in controlling both atrial and ventricular arrhythmias
    d. May induce parkinsonism
    e. Causes urinary retention

14. Theophylline—

    a. Induces the enzyme phosphodiesterase
    b. Has a positive inotropic effect on the heart
    c. Is largely excreted unchanged in the kidneys
    d. Causes fits at toxic levels
    e. Needs to be given in higher doses to smokers

15. Parkinsonism is an unwanted effect of—

    a. Phenytoin
    b. Chlorpromazine
    c. Baclofen
    d. Neostigmine
    e. Metoclopramide

Answers overleaf

11. a. False   Hepatocellular damage follows overdosage
     b. True   This causes a dose-related cholestasis, in common with oestrogens and anabolic steroids
     c. False
     d. True   Due to hypersensitivity reaction similar to that with chlorpromazine
     e. False   Haemolysis in association with glucose-6-phosphate dehydrogenase deficiency is the usual mechanism of jaundice

12. a. False   It is a mucopolysaccharide
     b. True
     c. False   It is about 2 hours
     d. False   Warfarin is secreted in breast milk
     e. True   Thrombocytopenia due to platelet destruction is a recognised side-effect

13. a. False   Like many antiarrhythmic agents it has a negative inotropic effect
     b. False   Although disopyramide may negate the positive inotropic effect of digoxin
     c. True
     d. False
     e. True   Due to its anticholinergic effect

14. a. False   The enzyme is inhibited
     b. True
     c. False   Only 7 per cent is excreted unchanged
     d. True
     e. True   Hepatic enzymes are induced in smokers

15. a. False   Phenytoin characteristically causes cerebellar signs
     b. True   It is a dopamine receptor blocker
     c. False
     d. False   It is an anticholinesterase
     e. True   It probably works in the same way as chlorpromazine

16. Beta-blocking agents that are highly water-soluble—

a. Are commonly associated with central nervous system side-effects
b. Are more likely to cause airways obstruction than lipid-soluble beta-blocking agents
c. Undergo extensive hepatic first pass metabolism
d. Require dose reduction in renal failure
e. Can usually be given once daily

17. Drugs that cause systemic lupus erythematosus include—

a. Procainamide
b. Gold
c. Phenytoin
d. Methotrexate
e. Isoniazid

18. Bromocriptine—

a. Causes retroperitoneal fibrosis
b. Decreases tumour size in prolactinomas
c. Alleviates symptoms of Raynaud's disease
d. Cause hypertension
e. Suppresses lactation

19. Hirsutism is a recognised side-effect of—

a. Spironolactone
b. Phenytoin
c. Cyclosporin
d. Digoxin
e. Clomiphene

20. Harmful interactions are likely with the use of—

a. Alcohol and metronidazole
b. Digoxin and nitrazepam
c. Warfarin and propranolol
d. Indomethacin and lithium
e. Salicylates and methotrexate

Answers overleaf

16. a. False These side-effects occur with lipid-soluble agents which cross the blood–brain barrier
　　b. False Cardioselectivity and lipid solubility are not directly related
　　c. False
　　d. True Predominantly renal clearance
　　e. True

17. a. True One of the most common causes along with hydrallazine and phenytoin
　　b. False
　　c. True As can other anticonvulsants including primidone and ethosuximide
　　d. False
　　e. True

18. a. True
　　b. True
　　c. False A dopamine agonist, it may aggravate vasospasm
　　d. False It is hypotensive
　　e. True

19. a. False It causes gynaecomastia
　　b. True
　　c. True
　　d. False
　　e. False Hair loss has been reported

20. a. True Metronidazole inhibits aldehyde dehydrogenase and causes a disulfiram-like reaction
　　b. False
　　c. False
　　d. True Indomethacin increases lithium concentrations
　　e. True Salicylates displace methotrexate from serum proteins

21. **Metronidazole is effective against—**

    a. *Actinomyces*
    b. *Bacteroides fragilis*
    c. *Staphylococcus aureus*
    d. *Entamoeba histolytica*
    e. *Clostridium welchii*

22. **Morphine—**

    a. Is conjugated in the liver
    b. Relaxes the gastro-oesophageal sphincter
    c. Causes peripheral vasodilatation
    d. Increases pressure in the sphincter of Oddi
    e. Causes urinary retention

23. **Drugs that are highly bound to plasma proteins (90 per cent or greater) include—**

    a. Cloxacillin
    b. Gentamicin
    c. Warfarin
    d. Chlorpromazine
    e. Digoxin

24. **Drugs with plasma half-lives of less than 12 hours include—**

    a. Amitriptyline
    b. Phenobarbitone
    c. Tolbutamide
    d. Ethosuximide
    e. Propranolol

25. **Penicillamine—**

    a. Is contraindicated in Still's disease
    b. May be safely restarted in some patients, once the platelet count has returned to normal, following an episode of thrombocytopenia
    c. Causes a reduction in the level of rheumatoid factor
    d. Is effective treatment in cystinuria
    e. Absorption is reduced when iron is given concurrently

Answers overleaf

21. a. False   The exception to the rule that it is effective against anaerobes
    b. True
    c. False
    d. True   It is also effective against *Giardia* and *Trichomonas*
    e. True

22. a. True
    b. False   In the gastrointestinal tract generally tone is increased while propulsive peristalsis is reduced
    c. True
    d. True
    e. True   By increasing sphincter tone, and by acting centrally to alter attention to bladder stimuli

23. a. True   Unlike other penicillins
    b. False   Neligible amounts are protein bound
    c. True
    d. True
    e. False

24. a. False   Over 24 hours and longer for the active metabolite
    b. False   80 hours
    c. True   5 hours. There is less risk of hypoglycaemia than with chlorpropamide
    d. False   Many antiepileptic agents have long half-lives and can be given once daily
    e. True   3 hours

25. a. False   It has been successfully used with the usual precautions
    b. True   Restart with a lower dose and increase slowly
    c. True
    d. True   Penicillamine binds cystine, forming a more soluble complex
    e. True   Iron is chelated in the gut and the complexes are not absorbed

Psychiatry

1. **In phobic disorders**

   a. Symptoms of anxiety are characteristic
   b. Males and females are affected with equal frequency
   c. Progressive disintegration of the personality occurs
   d. Exposure to the feared situation is used in treatment
   e. Antidepressant drugs are as effective as behavioural treatment

2. **Characteristic features of the neuroleptic malignant syndrome include—**

   a. Onset a few days after stopping phenothiazines
   b. Excessive salivation
   c. Hypotonia
   d. Hypothermia
   e. Raised serum creatine phosphokinase activity

3. **Characteristic features of anorexia nervosa include—**

   a. Hyperprolactinaemia
   b. Low levels of follicle stimulating hormone
   c. Low cholesterol concentration
   d. Low growth hormone concentration
   e. Hypokalaemia

4. **Factors that are associated with the development of anorexia nervosa include—**

   a. Delinquent behaviour in childhood
   b. Parents unemployed
   c. Family history of schizophrenia
   d. Thyroid dysfunction
   e. Large family size

5. **Characteristic features of childhood autism include—**

   a. Close relationship to parents
   b. Preoccupation with stereotyped routines
   c. Onset before the age of 5 years
   d. Intelligent quotient above 90
   e. Family history of schizophrenia

Answers overleaf

1. a. True
   b. False   Most phobias, e.g. agoraphobia (75%) and animal phobias (95%), are more common in women
   c. False
   d. True   Desensitisation by gradual introduction of the unpleasant situation is often used
   e. False   Behavioural treatments are the mainstay

2. a. False
   b. True   Disturbances of autonomic function are characteristic
   c. False   Muscle tone is increased
   d. False   Marked hyperthermia is characteristic
   e. True

3. a. False
   b. True   Levels of luteinising hormone are also low
   c. False   It is often increased
   d. False   It is often increased, as in any state of undernutrition
   e. True   Induced vomiting and laxative abuse may be responsible

4. a. False   Such children are often excessively good
   b. False
   c. False
   d. False   Various hormonal causes have been postulated but none proved. Bradycardia and low basal metabolic rate are a response to undernutrition and do not represent hypothyroidism
   e. False

5. a. False   Failure to form close emotional relationships is typical
   b. True
   c. True   It is rare after this age
   d. False   Majority have IQ below 70
   e. False   The idea that autism is a type of schizophrenia is out of fashion

6. **Mutism is a recognised feature of—**

    a. Alcohol withdrawal
    b. Conversion hysteria
    c. Catatonic schizophrenia
    d. Depression
    e. Ganser syndrome

7. **Depression is an unwanted effect of—**

    a. Indomethacin
    b. Methyldopa
    c. Temazepam
    d. Corticosteroids
    e. Captopril

8. **Characteristic features of obsessional states include—**

    a. Family history of schizophrenia
    b. Perseveration
    c. Onset in old age
    d. Good insight
    e. History of amphetamine abuse

9. **Disorientation in time is a characteristic feature of—**

    a. Korsakoff's psychosis
    b. Acute schizophrenic breakdown
    c. Hypomania
    d. Depressive psychosis
    e. Agoraphobia

10. **Echolalia is a recognised feature of—**

    a. Catatonic schizophrenia
    b. Gilles de la Tourette syndrome
    c. Alzheimer's disease
    d. Childhood autism
    e. Petit mal epilepsy

Answers overleaf

6. a. False
        b. True
        c. True
        d. True   In profound depressive stupor
        e. False This is a very rare condition, which may be a manifestation of hysteria. Approximate answers to questions are characteristic

7. a. True
        b. True   Probably by causing depletion of neurotransmitters
        c. False Generally depression is not a side-effect of benzodiazepine usage
        d. True
        e. False

8. a. False Although schizophrenics may have obsessions, they are a minority of those with obsessional disorders
        b. False This is a feature of dementia
        c. False Onset may be at any age but more often in the young
        d. True   They are usually all too aware of the problem
        e. False Amphetamine abuse can produce a psychosis

9. a. True   Short-term memory loss with confabulation is typical
        b. False
        c. False
        d. False
        e. False

10. a. True   A characteristic finding
        b. True   Other features include coprolalia and tics
        c. True
        d. True   Repetition of mannerisms and activities may also be seen
        e. False

11. **Characteristic features of schizophrenia include—**

    a. Obsessional thoughts
    b. Progression to dementia
    c. Delusions of guilt
    d. Early morning wakening
    e. Thought withdrawal

12. **Behaviour modification therapy is of use in—**

    a. Paedophilia
    b. Nocturnal enuresis
    c. Obsessional states
    d. Mania
    e. Agoraphobia

13. **In a patient with an acute schizophrenic breakdown a bad ultimate prognosis is suggested by—**

    a. Above average intelligence
    b. Flattening of affect
    c. Sudden onset
    d. Normal premorbid personality
    e. Family history of manic depression

14. **Risk factors for completed suicide include—**

    a. Being married
    b. Age under 20 years
    c. Alcoholism
    d. A history of having discussed suicide with a friend
    e. Severe, painful physical illness

15. **Severe mental subnormality is characteristic of—**

    a. Klinefelter's syndrome
    b. Lesch—Nyhan syndrome
    c. Neurofibromatosis
    d. Trisomy D
    e. Hurler's syndrome

Answers overleaf

11. a. False   They are sometimes seen, but are not character-istic

     b. False

     c. False   Characteristic of depressive psychosis

     d. False   A characteristic feature of depression

     e. True   A typical feature of schizophrenic thought dis-order

12. a. True   Extensive use of behaviour modification is made in treating various sexual problems

     b. True

     c. True   The environment can be gradually altered so that it is not possible for the obsessional act to be carried out

     d. False

     e. True   Perhaps the main use is in phobic disorders

13. a. False   The reverse is the case

     b. True

     c. False   This suggests a precipitating factor and, if this is removed, the patient may not relapse

     d. False

     e. False

14. a. False   The incidence is much higher in single, divorced or separated individuals

     b. False   Though attempted suicides are common

     c. True

     d. True

     e. True

15. a. False   Mild retardation is quite common

     b. True   A disorder of uric acid metabolism. The tendency to self-mutilation is particularly characteristic and distressing

     c. False

     d. True   Cardiac abnormalities and cleft palate are also characteristic

     e. True

16. Characteristic features of morphine withdrawal include—

    a. Excessive yawning
    b. Hypotension
    c. Muscle cramps
    d. Dry eyes
    e. Diarrhoea

17. In tardive dyskinesia—

    a. Metoclopramide is a recognised cause
    b. Intramuscular benztropine is rapidly effective in reversing the changes
    c. Facial grimacing is characteristic
    d. Intention tremor is a recognised sign
    e. Withdrawal of phenothiazines may precipitate an attack

18. Paranoid ideas are a recognised feature of—

    a. Delirium tremens
    b. Cancer phobia
    c. Depression
    d. Obsessional neurosis
    e. Dementia

19. Characteristic features of acute hypomania include—

    a. Retention of insight
    b. Flight of ideas
    c. Confabulation
    d. Distractability
    e. Family history of depression

20. Recognised features of depression include—

    a. Poor concentration
    b. Agitation
    c. Hypochondriasis
    d. Delusions of bodily influence
    e. Weight loss

Answers overleaf

16. a. True   One of the early features
    b. False Moderate hypertension is often seen
    c. True
    d. False Running eyes and rhinorrhoea are usual
    e. True

17. a. True
    b. False Treatment is difficult. Prevention by 'drug holi-
              days' has been suggested, where phenothiazines
              are stopped at regular intervals
    c. True
    d. False This is a sign of cerebellar disease
    e. True

18. a. True
    b. False
    c. True
    d. False
    e. True   Most causes of acute confusional states could
              also be responsible

19. a. False It is lost
    b. True
    c. False This is making up answers to cover a memory
              defect. It is characteristic of Korsakoff's psy-
              chosis
    d. True   These patients notice many things and can be
              easily set off on a different line of thought
    e. True   In bipolar illness (alternating mania and depres-
              sion) a family history is especially common

20. a. True   Mental processes are slowed though accuracy is
              usually preserved
    b. True
    c. True
    d. False A characteristic feature of schizophrenia
    e. True

Poisoning

1. Characteristic early features of salicylate poisoning in an adult include—

a. Coma
b. Acidosis
c. Tinnitus
d. Renal failure
e. Sweating

2. Recognised features of barbiturate poisoning include—

a. Liver necrosis
b. Hypotension
c. Hypothermia
d. Bullous rash
e. Reversal of respiratory depression by naloxone

3. In acute iron poisoning—

a. Delay in the onset of symptoms is recognised
b. Pyloric stenosis occurs as a late complication
c. Desferrioxamine acts so slowly that it is of little use
d. A history of paint spraying may be obtained
e. Liver necrosis is a complication

4. In acute paracetamol poisoning—

a. Loss of consciousness is characteristic
b. Those on long-term barbiturates are less severely affected
c. Acute tubular necrosis is a recognised complication
d. There is little risk if the patient survives the first 24 hours
e. Plasma concentration within 4 hours is a good predictor of liver damage

Answers overleaf

1. a. False   The patient is often awake and agitated. Coma
                tends to be late and serious
    b. False   Early on, alkalosis resulting from hyperventila-
                tion is the rule. Acidosis occurs later. In children
                acidosis may be present at an earlier stage
    c. True   Often one of the first signs of overdosage
    d. False   An occasional late complication
    e. True

2. a. False
    b. True   Due to a direct toxic effect on the myocardium as
                well as decreased venous return to the heart
                because of peripheral venous pooling
    c. True
    d. True   Glutethimide and tricyclic overdosage also cause
                bullous rashes
    e. False   Naloxone is used in opiate overdosage

3. a. True   Some hours may elapse
    b. True
    c. False   Given directly into the stomach and also paren-
                terally it chelates and removes useful amounts of
                iron
    d. False   Ingestion of iron-containing medication is the
                usual route of entry
    e. True   And may be fatal

4. a. False   It is uncommon unless other sedative drugs have
                also been taken
    b. False   Paracetamol is converted to a toxic metabolite in
                the liver, and this process will be increased if
                liver enzymes are already induced by barbi-
                turates
    c. True   Though liver necrosis is more common
    d. False   Liver necrosis may only become apparent after
                48 hours
    e. False   Absorption before 4 hours is likely to be in-
                complete

5. **Characteristic features of severe poisoning by the European adder (*Vipera berus*) include—**

    a. Severe hypotension
    b. Absence of local reaction to snake bite
    c. Neurotoxicity
    d. Neutrophil leucocytosis
    e. Abdominal pain

6. **In digoxin overdose—**

    a. Supraventricular tachycardia with variable atrioventricular block is characteristic
    b. Cholestyramine may reduce further digoxin absorption
    c. Forced diuresis increases drug elimination
    d. Administration of digoxin-specific antibody fragments increases renal clearance
    e. Hyperkalaemia is a recognised finding

Answers overleaf

5. a. True   This is a feature of severe poisoning but may also result from a vasovagal attack

    b. False   This can generally be taken to indicate that no poisoning has occurred

    c. False   This is a feature of bites with elapids (cobras) and sea snakes

    d. True

    e. True

6. a. True

    b. True

    c. False   Also peritoneal and haemodialysis do not significantly increase clearance of the drug

    d   True

    e. True   Due to inhibition of sodium and potassium activated ATPase enzyme systems

Renal Diseases

1. **Features in the nephrotic syndrome indicating a bad ultimate prognosis include—**

   a. Hyperlipidaemia
   b. Highly selective proteinuria
   c. Glomerular filtration rate of 10 ml per minute
   d. Proteinuria of greater than 10 g in 24 hours
   e. Onset in childhood

2. **Causes of renal papillary necrosis include—**

   a. Amyloidosis
   b. Penicillamine
   c. Sickle cell disease
   d. Renal tubular acidosis
   e. Diabetes mellitus

3. **A reduced serum complement level is characteristic of—**

   a. Minimal lesion glomerulonephritis
   b. Lupus nephritis
   c. Membranous glomerulonephritis
   d. Acute post-streptococcal glomerulonephritis
   e. Mesangiocapillary glomerulonephritis

4. **Causes of hypokalaemia include—**

   a. Addison's disease
   b. Gentamicin
   c. Chronic pyelonephritis
   d. Diabetes insipidus
   e. Bronchial carcinoma

Answers overleaf

1 a. False This is generally of no prognostic significance. Nephrotic syndrome due to systemic lupus is said not to give hyperlipidaemia

    b. False

    c. True If renal failure of this degree has developed the outlook would generally be poor

    d. False

    e. False Minimal lesion glomerulonephritis with a relatively good prognosis is common in childhood

2. a. False

    b. False Analgesic drugs may be responsible

    c. True Ischaemia is caused by sludging of red cells in the renal papillae

    d. False

    e. True May present chronically as is usual with other causes of papillary necrosis, or sometimes acutely in association with severe infection

3. a. False

    b. True

    c. False Though complement is deposited in the glomeruli in this and many other renal disease, complement production often enables the serum level to remain normal

    d. True

    e. True A profound hypocomplementaemia is usual

4. a. False Hyperkalaemia is usual

    b. True

    c. True Potassium loss is occasionally marked

    d. False

    e. True Due to ectopic ACTH production

5. **A patient has suffered considerable blood loss and has been oliguric for some hours. Factors that point towards acute tubular necrosis which will not be reversed by fluid replacement include an increase in—**

   a. Blood urea
   b. Urinary sodium excretion
   c. Urinary urea excretion
   d. Urinary osmolarity
   e. Urine volume

6. **A strongly acid urine is a recognised feature of—**

   a. Severe pyloric stenosis
   b. Renal tubular acidosis
   c. Chronic obstructive airways disease
   d. Chronic renal failure
   e. Urinary tract infection with *Proteus*

7. **Features that suggest the presence of underlying chronic renal failure in a patient with acute renal failure include—**

   a. Bilateral small kidneys on pyelography
   b. Renal osteodystrophy
   c. Reduced plasma bicarbonate concentration
   d. Raised serum phosphate concentration
   e. Normocytic normochromic anaemia

8. **An elevated blood urea level is characteristic of—**

   a. Severe pyloric stenosis
   b. Nephrotic syndrome
   c. Excessive antidiuretic hormone secretion
   d. Liver cirrhosis
   e. Gastrointestinal haemorrhage

Answers overleaf

5. a. False   Any cause of extracellular fluid volume depletion will increase the blood urea

    b. True   In tubular necrosis sodium is not reabsorbed

    c. False   In tubular necrosis excretion of urea is not reduced

    d. False   In tubular necrosis the osmolarity falls due to failure to concentrate urine, while in volume depletion the urine is keenly concentrated

    e. False   Oliguria should persist

6. a. True   The severe fluid depletion causes sodium reabsorption (with loss of hydrogen and potassium ions) to override acid–base considerations. Since potassium is already low hydrogen ion is lost at the distal tubule despite the systemic alkalosis

    b. False   Failure to produce an acid urine is the problem

    c. True   In an attempt to compensate for the respiratory acidosis

    d. True   Despite an overall reduction in hydrogen ion excretion and systemic acidosis. The mechanism of acid urine is obscure

    e. False   *Proteus* splits urea, resulting in production of ammonia

7. a. True   Small kidneys are typical of chronic glomerulonephritis and chronic pyelonephritis

    b. True

    c. False   Acidosis occurs in acute and chronic renal failure

    d. False   Again this occurs in both acute and chronic renal failure

    e. True   Anaemia takes time to develop

8. a. True   Due to dehydration

    b. False   Renal failure is not necessarily a feature of nephrotic syndrome

    c. False   Haemodilution occurs

    d. False   Urea is low due to failure of liver synthesis

    e. True   Due to ingestion of a large amount of protein from breakdown of blood

9. **Characteristic features of the nephrotic syndrome include—**

   a. Increased plasma volume
   b. Hyperlipidaemia
   c. Reduced urinary sodium excretion
   d. Bence-Jones protein in the urine
   e. Leuconychia

10. **There is a characteristic association between high renin levels and—**

    a. Conn's syndrome
    b. Addison's disease
    c. Propranolol therapy
    d. Increased potassium intake
    e. Captopril

11. **Causes of hyperchloraemic acidosis include—**

    a. Diabetic ketoacidosis
    b. Ureterosigmoidostomy
    c. Renal tubular acidosis
    d. Chronic obstructive airways disease
    e. Acute glomerulonephritis

12. **A clinical picture of acute nephritis is a well-recognised feature of—**

    a. Minimal change glomerulonephritis
    b. Polyarteritis nodosa
    c. Renal vein thrombosis
    d. Diabetes mellitus
    e. Membranous glomerulonephritis

13. **Characteristic features of Alport's syndrome (hereditary nephritis) include—**

    a. Autosomal recessive inheritance
    b. Heavy proteinuria
    c. Frank haematuria
    d. Response to steroid therapy at high dose
    e. Earlier onset of clinical features in males

Answers overleaf

9. a. False   The intravascular volume is reduced due to loss
                 of fluid from the hypoalbuminaemic circulation.
                 This induces hyperaldosteronism and retention
                 of fluid, which in turn is lost from the circulation
                 to become tissue oedema
    b. True
    c. True   Due to the secondary hyperaldosteronism
    d. False
    e. True   As with other hypoalbuminaemic states

10. a. False   Increased aldosterone is the primary event and
                 this lowers renin by negative feedback
    b. True   The low sodium and low renal perfusion pressure
                 elevate renin
    c. False   The sympathetic nervous system causes renin
                 release
    d. False   Renin concentrations are reduced
    e. True

11. a. False   Various unmeasured anions constitute an 'anion
                 gap'
    b. True   Due to exchange of bicarbonate for chloride
                 across the intestinal epithelium
    c. True   Systemic acidosis is due to an inability to produce
                 an acid urine. Chloride increases to fill the anion
                 gap
    d. False   A compensated respiratory acidosis is usual
    e. False

12. a. False   It usually presents as nephrotic syndrome
    b. True   Nephritis also occurs in other vasculitic disorders
    c. False   Usually associated with nephrotic syndrome
    d. False
    e. False   Though it may present with haematuria, an acute
                 fulminating course is not a feature

13. a. False   Dominant (autosomal or X-linked)
    b. False   Proteinuria is usually light and nephrotic syn-
                 drome rare
    c. True   Usual presenting feature
    d. False
    e. True

14. **Recognised features of renal tubular acidosis include—**

    a. Systemic alkalosis
    b. Hypokalaemia
    c. Repeated urinary tract infection
    d. Nephrocalcinosis
    e. Hypochloraemia

15. **A woman in end-stage renal failure who starts regular haemo-dialysis can confidently expect—**

    a. Anaemia to improve
    b. To avoid developing renal bone disease
    c. To observe no fluid restriction
    d. Nausea and vomiting to improve
    e. Return of fertility

Answers overleaf

14. a. False There is acidosis
    b. True Potassium is lost at the distal tubule instead of hydrogen ions, which cannot be excreted
    c. True
    d. True Associated with hypercalciuria
    e. False Chloride levels are elevated to fill the anion gap left by low bicarbonate concentration

15. a. False Occasionally it does, but not usually. It may be worsened by leakage of blood, and further reduction in erythropoietin if bilateral nephrectomy is done
    b. False As patients do not die from uraemia, metabolic bone problems may become more apparent
    c. False After onset of dialysis urinary output may fall and fluid restriction must be observed if heart failure and hypertension are to be avoided
    d. True Where these are due to uraemia
    e. False While libido and periods may return, fertility rarely does

Respiratory Medicine

1. Causes of massive haemoptysis include—

a. Bronchiectasis
b. Tuberculosis
c. Chronic bronchitis
d. Aspergilloma
e. Systemic lupus erythematosus

2. Causes of finger clubbing include—

a. Simple coal workers' pneumoconiosis
b. Chronic bronchitis
c. Ulcerative colitis
d. Addison's disease
e. Mesothelioma of the pleura

3. Hypertrophic pulmonary osteoarthropathy is associated with—

a. Gynaecomastia
b. Periosteal new bone formation
c. Bronchial neoplasia, usually of oat cell type
d. Alleviation by vagotomy
e. Bone pain

4. A man 60 years old has bronchial carcinoma. Attempts at curative resection are contraindicated if he has—

a. Hilar adenopathy demonstrated on computed tomography
b. Forced expiratory volume in 1 second of 2 litres
c. Superior vena caval syndrome
d. Pleural effusion
e. Sensorimotor neuropathy

Answers overleaf

1. a. True The quantity of haemoptysis is not a reliable guide to causation, but there are few causes of massive haemoptysis

    b. True A cavity may erode a branch of the pulmonary artery. Bleeding can be fatal

    c. False Haemoptysis if it occurs is slight and other causes should always be excluded

    d. True

    e. False Haemoptysis is a recognised feature but is usually slight

2. a. False

    b. False Some might dispute this, but 'false' is the safe answer

    c. True Other diseases such as Crohn's disease, malabsorption and liver cirrhosis also cause it

    d. False

    e. True

3. a. True Probably due to gonadotrophin formation

    b. True This can be seen on X-rays of wrists and ankles

    c. False Finger clubbing and hypertrophic pulmonary osteoarthropathy are more often seen with squamous carcinomas

    d. True Excision of the tumour or steroids may also help

    e. True

4. a. False Local hilar adenopathy does not contraindicate surgery, but mediastinal node enlargement may do so

    b. False The generally accepted minimum FEV_1 is 1 litre, although other pulmonary function data should be taken into account

    c. True This implies local extension

    d. False The effusion may be secondary to obstructive pneumonitis. Malignant cells in the effusion or on pleural biopsy should be sought

    e. False This is a non-metastatic manifestation

5. Bronchial carcinoids—

    a. Occur more frequently in smokers
    b. Can usually be resected endoscopically
    c. May present with a lung abscess
    d. May give rise to valve lesions of the left side of the heart
    e. Can be locally invasive

6. In pulmonary alveolar proteinosis—

    a. Alveoli contain substance rich in phospholipid
    b. Haemoptysis is a recognised feature
    c. Pleural effusions occur
    d. Pulmonary lavage using several litres of fluid is helpful
    e. Steroids prevent deterioration in lung function

7. A boy 18 years old has a moderately severe attack of asthma. One would expect to find—

    a. Po_2 less than 60 mmHg (8.0 kPa)
    b. Pco_2 greater than 60 mmHg (8.0 kPa)
    c. Raised plasma bicarbonate level
    d. Immediate relief by intravenous injection of hydrocortisone
    e. Dehydration

8. An exacerbation of farmer's lung—

    a. Is more common in summer
    b. Is characterised by intense wheeze
    c. Produces eosinophilia in the peripheral blood
    d. Is excluded by the absence of precipitating antibodies
    e. Usually responds to steroids

9. Mesothelioma of the pleura—

    a. May follow asbestos exposure 30 years previously
    b. Characteristically develops on a pleural plaque
    c. Is a Prescribed Disease
    d. May produce a chest X-ray resembling a pleural effusion
    e. Is slowly progressive over many years following diagnosis

Answers overleaf

5. a. False
    b. False   Usually only the 'tip of the iceberg' can be seen through the bronchoscope
    c. True   By bronchial obstruction
    d. True   They produce 5-hydroxy-tryptamine, which is released into the pulmonary venous circulation and hence reaches the left side of the heart. With carcinoids from other sites the active peptides are broken down in the lungs
    e. True

6. a. True   Gives a diffuse, finely nodular appearance on chest radiograph
    b. False   Exertional dyspnoea and mucoid sputum are the characteristic features
    c. False
    d. True
    e. False

7. a. True
    b. False   Generally carbon dioxide is adequately excreted. If retention occurs artificial ventilation should be considered
    c. False   In respiratory acidosis with carbon dioxide retention such a compensatory metabolic change occurs, for example in chronic bronchitis
    d. False   It takes a few hours
    e. True   It may need correction with intravenous fluids

8. a. False   It occurs when mouldy stored hay is used for winter feeding
    b. False   Airways obstruction is not a prominent feature
    c. False   This is characteristic of asthma
    d. False   These are not found in some typical cases
    e. True

9. a. True   Such cases occur
    b. False   No obvious relation to pleural plaques is recognised
    c. True   And compensation is available
    d. True
    e. False

10. **Characteristic features of silicosis include—**

    a. Worsening of symptoms when returning to work after a few days off
    b. Predisposition to tuberculosis
    c. Exertional dyspnoea
    d. Response to steroids
    e. Focal fibrosis of the lower lobes

11. **Features of idiopathic pulmonary haemosiderosis include—**

    a. Recurrent haemoptysis
    b. Onset in those over 50 years of age
    c. Hypochromic anaemia
    d. Haemosiderin-laden macrophages in the sputum
    e. Satisfactory response to desferrioxamine

12. **In a patient with seropositive rheumatoid arthritis, findings on examination of pleural fluid aspirate that would point to a cause for the effusion other than rheumatoid disease are—**

    a. 120,000 red cells per mm^3
    b. Glucose concentration 1.2 mmol/l
    c. pH 7.15
    d. 20,000 white cells per mm^3
    e. Lactate dehydrogenase 180 i.u./l (normal serum concentration 120–400 i.u./l)

13. **A single 3-cm rounded shadow outside the hilum on chest X-ray with no other abnormality could be due to—**

    a. Hydatid disease
    b. Secondary carcinoma
    c. Sarcoidosis
    d. Wegener's granulomatosis
    e. Pulmonary alveolar proteinosis

14. **Features of occupational asbestos exposure include—**

    a. A restrictive lung defect
    b. More severe lung disease when many asbestos bodies are found in the sputum
    c. Non-malignant pleural effusion
    d. Lung nodules
    e. Calcified pleural plaques

Answers overleaf

10. a. False This is characteristic of byssinosis
     b. True   This should always be suspected if a rapid deterioration occurs
     c. True
     d. False
     e. False The focal fibrosis tends to affect the upper lobes

11. a. True
     b. False It is more common in young people
     c. True   Due to blood loss from haemoptysis
     d. True   Although characteristic they are by no means specific
     e. False Overall iron overload is not a problem

12. a. True   Would raise suspicion of malignancy or pulmonary infarct
     b. False Low glucose concentration and pH are characteristic
     c. False
     d. True
     e. True   Usually elevated in rheumatoid effusion

13. a. True
     b. True
     c. False Masses due to lymph nodes may occur in the hilum
     d. True
     e. False This rare disease is characterised by a diffuse infiltration of the alveoli with a lipoprotein

14. a. True
     b. False Asbestos bodies only indicate exposure to asbestos, and do not by themselves indicate lung changes
     c. True   Caused by inflammation of the pleura
     d. False Fibrotic changes are diffuse affecting especially the lower lobes
     e. True   But these do not correlate with changes in the lung parenchyma

15. In emphysema the following parameters of lung function are reduced—

    a. Ratio of forced expiratory volume in 1 second to forced vital capacity

    b. Residual volume

    c. Peak flow rate

    d. Lung compliance

    e. Transfer factor for carbon monoxide (T_{LCO})

16. In pneumonia due to *Mycoplasma pneumoniae*—

    a. Malaise and headaches are common presenting symptoms

    b. Radiological changes lag behind the physical signs

    c. Pleural effusion is a common complication

    d. Cold agglutinins are found in over 80 per cent of cases

    e. Stevens–Johnson syndrome is a recognised association

17. Recognised findings in sarcoidosis include—

    a. Bilateral facial nerve palsy

    b. Haemolytic anaemia

    c. Erythema multiforme

    d. Heart block

    e. Lacrimal gland enlargement

18. Causes of diffuse lung fibrosis include—

    a. Byssinosis

    b. Rheumatoid arthritis

    c. Pneumococcal pneumonia

    d. Bleomycin

    e. Goodpasture's syndrome·

Answers overleaf

15. a. True   Emphysema causes airways obstruction
     b. False It is increased due to air trapping
     c. True   Again due to airways obstruction
     d. False There is loss of elastic tissue and therefore the lung volume will change more easily for a given pressure change
     e. True   Although we think of transfer factor as a measure of diffusion being characteristically depressed in diseases affecting the alveolus (such as fibrosing alveolitis), it is also affected by ventilation/perfusion abnormalities. It is better to think of it as a measure of overall gas exchange and this is impaired in emphysema

16. a. True   As in other non-bacterial pneumonias
     b. False The reverse is the case
     c. False A rare complication
     d. False Present in approximately 50 per cent of cases, but often looked for to help make a diagnosis
     e. True   Also erythema multiforme alone

17. a. True   It may be part of Heerfordt's syndrome, which also includes parotitis and uveitis
     b. False
     c. False Erythema nodosum, lupus pernio and a generalised nodular or papular eruption are the usual skin manifestations
     d. True   Due to sarcoid granulomas affecting the conducting system
     e. True

18. a. False In the chronic stages of byssinosis, bronchitis and emphysema occur but no fibrosis
     b. True   As with other connective tissue disorders
     c. False
     d. True   As with a long list of other drugs
     e. True   Pulmonary haemorrhage occurs and lung fibrosis may ensue

19. Pneumothorax is a recognised complication of—

    a. Pulmonary infarction
    b. Staphylococcal pneumonia
    c. Ehlers–Danlos syndrome
    d. Tuberculosis
    e. Pleural mesothelioma

20. In aspirin-sensitive asthma—

    a. There is a type 1 hypersensitivity reaction to salicylates
    b. Females are more commonly affected than males
    c. Non-steroidal anti-inflammatory drugs can safely be given
    d. Eosinophilia is common
    e. Altered arachidonic acid metabolism is the underlying mechanism

21. In a 25-year-old patient, who has started rifampicin, isoniazid and pyrazinamide for pulmonary tuberculosis—

    a. Coexistence of mild chronic renal failure should lead to reduction in dosage of rifampicin
    b. Development of peripheral neuropathy after 3 months' therapy will be reversed by administration of thiamine
    c. A standard combined contraceptive pill will be metabolised more rapidly than normal
    d. An acute attack of gout should lead to the substitution of isoniazid with an alternative drug
    e. The development of a syndrome of restlessness, insomnia and confusion should lead to the substitution of pyrazinamide with an alternative drug

22. Conditions predisposing to bronchiectasis include—

    a. Rubella infection in childhood
    b. Hypogammaglobulinaemia
    c. Kartagener's syndrome
    d. Carbon monoxide poisoning
    e. Hypothyroidism

Answers overleaf

19. a. False
   b. True
   c. True   Connective tissue is abnormal. Small subpleural cysts occur and may rupture
   d. True
   e. False

20. a. False
   b. True   Roughly twice as common
   c. False   In some individuals bronchospasm may also occur with these drugs
   d. False
   e. True   Aspirin blocks cyclo-oxygenase pathways and increased leukotrienes are produced by the lipo-oxygenase pathway

21. a. False   Rifampicin is excreted through the biliary system
   b. False   Pyridoxine prevents the peripheral neuropathy induced by isoniazid
   c. True   And contraceptive effectiveness is reduced
   d. False   Pyrazinamide causes hyperuricaemia
   e. False   Psychosis is an occasional side-effect of isoniazid

22. a. False   But measles and whooping cough are important causes
   b. True
   c. True   Immotile cilia fail to clear bronchial secretions
   d. False
   e. False

23. Calcification of the pleura on chest radiograph may be due to—

    a. Byssinosis
    b. Siderosis
    c. Previous haemothorax
    d. Chickenpox
    e. Mitral valve disease

24. In staphylococcal pneumonia—

    a. Consolidation on chest radiograph is often bilateral
    b. Emphysema as a complication is more common in adults than children
    c. Symptoms develop insidiously
    d. Bacterial resistance to flucloxacillin is common
    e. Pneumatocoele is a recognised complication

25. Features of Legionnaires' disease include—

    a. Raised serum creatinine concentration
    b. Most severe course in young, fit individuals
    c. Lymphocytosis
    d. Peak incidence in summer
    e. Mental confusion

Answers overleaf

23. a. False
   b. False
   c. True Asbestos exposure and previous tuberculous emphysema are other causes
   d. False Nodular parenchymal calcification may follow chickenpox pneumonitis
   e. False Nodular lung calcification is a rare complication of longstanding pulmonary oedema due to mitral valve disease

24. a. True Homogeneous or patchy
   b. False Emphysema and pleural effusion are both much more common in children
   c. False Rapid deterioration with death in hours is the danger of this condition
   d. False This is standard therapy, alone or with fusidic acid
   e. True Also pneumothorax

25. a. True
   b. False Fatality occurs in the old and infirm
   c. False A neutrophil leucocytosis with lymphopenia is usual
   d. True
   e. True

Rheumatology

1. **Characteristic features of Reiter's disease include—**

   a. Cutaneous vasculitis
   b. Pericarditis
   c. Scleromalacia
   d. Sacroiliitis
   e. Eosinophilia

2. **Characteristic features of polymyalgia rheumatica include—**

   a. Raised creatine kinase levels
   b. Response to steroids within a few days
   c. Abnormal electromyogram
   d. Normocytic anaemia
   e. Morning stiffness

3. **Hyperuricaemia is found in—**

   a. Chronic myeloid leukaemia
   b. Psoriasis
   c. Low-dose salicylate administration
   d. Starvation
   e. Xanthinuria

4. **Mouth ulcers are a recognised feature of—**

   a. Psoriasis
   b. Hyperthyroidism
   c. Crohn's disease
   d. Reiter's disease
   e. Coeliac disease

5. **Features more characteristic of the drug-induced form of systemic lupus than other cases of systemic lupus include—**

   a. Equal sex incidence
   b. Kidney involvement
   c. Fatal outcome
   d. Low complement levels
   e. Antibodies to native double-stranded DNA

Answers overleaf

1.   a. False   This is characteristic of seropositive arthritis
     b. False   Again a feature of seropositive arthritis
     c. False   Conjunctivitis and iritis are the usual eye changes in Reiter's disease
     d. True   As with all seronegative arthritis
     e. False

2.   a. False   Muscle enzymes are usually normal
     b. True   Diagnostic in itself
     c. False
     d. True
     e. True

3.   a. True   As with many haematological and other malignancies
     b. True
     c. True   At higher doses proximal tubular reabsorption of urate is reduced
     d. True
     e. False   Due to absence of xanthine oxidase, uric acid is not produced

4.   a. False
     b. False
     c. True
     d. True
     e. True   Other causes include simple aphthous ulceration, trauma, folate deficiency and Behçet's syndrome

5.   a. True   In other cases females are much more commonly affected
     b. False
     c. False   Recovery after stopping the offending drug often occurs
     d. False
     e. False

6. **Characteristic features of systemic sclerosis include—**

   a. Long-term benefit of corticosteroids
   b. Oesophageal stricture
   c. Obstructive ventilatory defect
   d. Asymmetrical polyarthritis
   e. Telangiectasia

7. **Features of ankylosing spondylitis include—**

   a. Presentation with polyarthritis
   b. Apical lung fibrosis
   c. Osteophytes on X-ray of lumbar spine
   d. Aortic incompetence
   e. Sciatica

8. **Features recognised as normal in joint fluid include—**

   a. Low viscosity
   b. Cell count of $0.2 \times 10^9/l$ (200 per mm^3)
   c. Glucose level half that of blood
   d. Presence of fibrin clot
   e. A few crystals of hydroxyapatite

9. **Recognised skin manifestations of dermatomyositis include—**

   a. Squamous carcinoma of the skin
   b. Yellow nails
   c. Periorbital oedema
   d. Nail fold haemorrhages
   e. Xanthomas

10. **In a patient with symmetrical polyarthritis, features that would point towards a diagnosis of systemic lupus erythematosus (SLE) as opposed to rheumatoid arthritis include—**

    a. Positive Coombs' test
    b. Subperiosteal erosions
    c. Livedo reticularis
    d. Antiphospholipid antibodies
    e. Recurrent pulmonary embolism

Answers overleaf

6. a. False   No effect is proved
     b. True
     c. False   A restrictive lung defect is usual
     d. False   Symmetrical polyarthritis is usual
     e. True

7. a. True   It may resemble rheumatoid arthritis
     b. True   And is occasionally complicated by cavitation
     c. False   Syndesmophytes are the typical finding
     d. True
     e. False

8. a. False   It is normally high due to hyaluronic acid
     b. True
     c. False   This would suggest septic or tuberculous arthritis
     d. False   None should be present as normal fluid does not contain fibrinogen
     e. False   Crystals are not normally present

9. a. False   The association is with internal malignancy
     b. False   Classically seen in the yellow nail syndrome, which is associated with lymphoedema
     c. True   Associated with the typical heliotrope rash
     d. True
     e. False

10. a. True   It is found in 15 per cent of patients with SLE. It is rare in rheumatoid arthritis
     b. False   Erosive arthritis is less common in SLE
     c. True
     d. True   A feature of SLE
     e. True   A well-recognised feature of SLE

11. Punched-out lesions on X-ray of the hands are recognised in—

a. Marfan's syndrome
b. Hypertrophic pulmonary osteoarthropathy
c. Gout
d. Sarcoid
e. Brucellosis

12. Joints involved more characteristically in rheumatoid arthritis than osteoarthritis include—

a. First carpometacarpal joint of the hand
b. Acromioclavicular joint
c. Cricoarytenoid
d. Wrists
e. Apophyseal joints of the lower cervical vertebrae

13. A polyarthropathy is a recognised feature of—

a. Acromegaly
b. Thyrotoxicosis
c. Sarcoidosis
d. Wilson's disease
e. Infectious hepatitis

14. Anti-Ro autoantibodies are commonly found in serum in—

a. Polymyalgia rheumatica
b. Sjögren's syndrome
c. Wegener's granulomatosis
d. Patients with a history of recurrent abortion and vascular thrombosis
e. Patients with features of lupus erythematosus and negative antinuclear antibody

Answers overleaf

11. a. False   Arachnodactyly may be noticed
     b. False   Periosteal new bone formation at the wrists and ankles is typical
     c. True
     d. True   They do not usually cause symptoms but tend to be associated with skin sarcoid
     e. False   Occasionally X-ray changes are seen in the spine

12. a. False   This is typical of osteoarthritis
     b. False   Again typical of osteoarthritis
     c. True
     d. True   Not commonly affected in osteoarthritis unless as a sequel to injury
     e. False   Rheumatoid arthritis tends to affect the upper cervical spine

13. a. True   A symmetrical polyarthropathy may be seen
     b. False   But occurs in myxoedema
     c. True   An acute polyarthropathy may be seen with erythema nodosum, but a chronic form also occurs
     d. False   As there are a great number of rare causes of polyarthropathy it can be hard to have courage and put 'false'
     e. True   Other rarer causes of polyarthropathy to remember include haemochromatosis, hyperparathyroidism, hyperlipidaemia and many acute infections

14. a. False
     b. True
     c. False   Antineutrophil cytoplasmic antibody is often present
     d. False   Antiphospholipid (cardiolipin) antibody is associated with these problems
     e. True

15. Features of polyarteritis nodosa include—

    a. Focal glomerulonephritis
    b. More common in females
    c. Positive hepatitis B surface antigen
    d. Myocardial infarction
    e. Polymorph leucocytosis

Answers overleaf

15. a. True
   b. False Unlike the other collagen diseases it is more common in males
   c. True Positive in 30 per cent of classic polyarteritis nodosa cases
   d. True The coronary arteries may be involved
   e. True Eosinophilia is often mentioned, but less common

Sexually Transmitted Diseases

1. **Characteristic features of secondary syphilis include—**

   a. Mucosal erosions
   b. Painless lymphadenopathy
   c. Severe constitutional features
   d. Interstitial keratitis
   e. Itchy rash

2. **The fluorescent treponemal antibody test is characteristically positive—**

   a. In yaws
   b. In glandular fever
   c. Within 3 weeks of infection with *Treponema pallidum*
   d. In tabes dorsalis
   e. In secondary syphilis

3. **Characteristic features of acute gonococcal urethritis in males include—**

   a. Incubation period of around 14 days
   b. High fever
   c. Response to tetracycline
   d. Reliable diagnosis by serology
   e. Genital ulceration

4. **Lymphogranuloma venereum—**

   a. Is endemic throughout the USA
   b. May be complicated by urethral stricture
   c. Is characterised by massive penile ulceration
   d. Erythema nodosum is a recognised feature
   e. Is best treated with penicillin

5. **Sexually transmitted diseases that are associated with arthritis include—**

   a. Gonorrhoea
   b. *Trichomonas vaginalis* infection
   c. Non-specific urethritis
   d. Lymphogranuloma venereum
   e. Syphilis

Answers overleaf

1. a. True
　　b. True
　　c. False　The generalised illness is usually mild
　　d. False　This is characteristic of congenital syphilis. Iritis is the main but uncommon eye complication of secondary syphilis
　　e. False　The rash is non-irritant

2. a. True　Syphilitic serology does not distinguish between *Treponema pallidum* and other treponemal strains
　　b. False　Although a transient positive Wassermann reaction occurs
　　c. False　Although the test is the first to become positive, this is still too early
　　d. True
　　e. True　Serology should be positive by this stage

3. a. False　2–8 days
　　b. False
　　c. True　Tetracycline will also be effective against some of the organisms of non-gonococcal urethritis
　　d. False　Standard serological tests do not distinguish an acute attack from previous infection
　　e. False　This would suggest coexistence of another sexually acquired disease

4. a. False　Although venereal disease is common in the USA, lymphogranuloma venereum is rare, and usually imported from abroad
　　b. True　Although rectal stricture is characteristic
　　c. False　The initial penile lesion may escape notice. Later inguinal lymphadenopathy may ulcerate
　　d. True
　　e. False　It is only slightly penicillin-sensitive

5. a. True
　　b. False
　　c. True
　　d. False　Causes arthralgia
　　e. True

6. Acquired immune deficiency syndrome (AIDS) is associated with—

    a.   Hypogammaglobulinaemia
    b.   Raised concentrations of β_2-microglobulin
    c.   Anergy to delayed hypersensitivity skin testing
    d.   Lymphocytosis
    e.   Antibody to P24 antigen

Answers overleaf

6. a. False Hypergammaglobulinaemia
 b. True Useful prognostic indicator
 c. True
 d. False Lymphopenia with selective deficiency of the helper T-cell subset is characteristic
 e. True Basis of ELISA test for HIV antibody

Symptoms and Signs

1. **Causes of palmar erythema include—**

   a. Rheumatoid arthritis
   b. Pregnancy
   c. Hypopituitarism
   d. Multiple sclerosis
   e. Thyrotoxicosis

2. **Extensor plantars and absent ankle jerks are a feature of—**

   a. Tabes dorsalis
   b. Friedreich's ataxia
   c. Multiple sclerosis
   d. Parasagittal meningioma
   e. Vitamin B_{12} deficiency

3. **Causes of splinter haemorrhages include—**

   a. Trauma
   b. Hypothyroidism
   c. Trichinosis
   d. Sarcoidosis
   e. Severe rheumatoid arthritis

4. **Increased skin sweating is a feature of—**

   a. Acromegaly
   b. Cystic fibrosis
   c. Anxiety
   d. Heat stroke
   e. Atropine poisoning

5. **Typical findings in a patient with Holmes–Adie (myotonic) pupil are—**

   a. Presentation in childhood
   b. Sluggish reaction to light and slow redilatation
   c. Constriction in response to pilocarpine
   d. Affected pupil larger than normal
   e. Extensor plantars

Answers overleaf

1. a. True
   b. True Excessive oestrogen is also the probable mechanism in liver failure
   c. False
   d. False
   e. True Chronic febrile illness and chronic leukaemias are the other causes which are quoted

2. a. False Tabes affects the dorsal columns and roots and would cause loss of ankle jerks by interrupting the sensory side of the reflex arc. Coexistent general paresis would be required to give the upper motor defect of extensor plantars
   b. True
   c. False
   d. False This is a cause of spastic paraplegia
   e. True A combination of peripheral neuropathy and subacute combined degeneration

3. a. True A much more common cause than infective endocarditis
   b. False
   c. True
   d. False
   e. True They are also found in some skin diseases. Rare causes quoted are malignant neoplasm and mitral stenosis

4. a. True
   b. False Though the electrolyte content of sweat is abnormal
   c. True
   d. False Loss of capacity to sweat is one of the problems
   e. False Atropine blocks the cholinergic stimulus of normal sweating

5. a. False Usually an incidental finding in young adults
   b. True
   c. True Denervation hypersensitivity
   d. True Occasionally smaller
   e. False Occasionally knee and ankle reflexes are absent

6. **Onycholysis is characteristic of—**

   a. Thyrotoxicosis
   b. Psoriasis
   c. Fungal infection of the nails
   d. Syphilis
   e. Nephrotic syndrome

7. **Increased melanin pigmentation is a recognised feature of—**

   a. Primary biliary cirrhosis
   b. Chédiak–Higashi syndrome
   c. Haemochromatosis
   d. Renal failure
   e. Hyperthyroidism

8. **A diastolic murmur of mitral origin may be due to—**

   a. Atrial septal defect
   b. Hypertrophic obstructive cardiomyopathy
   c. Patent ductus arteriosus
   d. Aortic incompetence
   e. Fallot's tetralogy

9. **Recognised causes of Raynaud's phenomenon include—**

   a. Carcinoid syndrome
   b. Scleroderma
   c. Cervical rib
   d. Cryoglobulinaemia
   e. Psoriasis

10. **Erythema nodosum occurs in association with—**

    a. Leprosy
    b. Crohn's disease
    c. Diabetes mellitus
    d. Penicillin therapy
    e. Internal malignancy

Answers overleaf

6. a. True   It also occurs in hypothyroidism, though less
often
   b. True
   c. True   Trauma is the other common cause. Others are
idiopathic
   d. False
   e. False   Leuconychia is seen

7. a. True   Melanin pigmentation may be early. Hyperbili-
rubinaemia may also contribute to skin colour
   b. False   Depigmentation is characteristic
   c. True   Iron may also contribute
   d. True   Urochrome also contributes
   e. True   As with a number of other endocrine disorders,
e.g. Addison's disease

8. a. False   A tricuspid diastolic murmur may be heard due
to increased flow
   b. False   The basic murmur is due to aortic outflow obstruction. Mitral incompetence is common later
   c. True   Due to increased flow
   d. True   Probably due to vibration of the anterior cusp by
the regurgitant aortic jet (Austin Flint murmur)
   e. False

9. a. False   Facial flushing is characteristic
   b. True   Other collagen diseases are also associated
   c. True   And other causes of vascular occlusion
   d. True   And other dysproteinaemias
   e. False   Do not forget Raynaud's disease, vibrating tools
and drugs as other causes

10. a. True   And in response to other infections
   b. True   Also ulcerative colitis
   c. False
   d. True
   e. True

Index

Index

Index